Single Port 11mm Laparoscopic Hysterectomy

(LESS-11mm)

An Advanced Ultra-Minimally Invasive Surgical Technique

By: Greg J. Marchand MD, FACS, FICS, FACOG

Disclosures / Conflicts of Interest

I have no conflicts of interest and nothing to declare.

Think about that for a minute.

All these devices mentioned — all this work and all this expert use of expensive surgical equipment — and no product representative even bought me dinner or invited me to their speaker board?

Fuck...did I get shafted or what?

Completed text found exempt from review at IRB - August 2019.

ISBN: 0-578-56875-1
ISBN-13: 978-0-578-56875-1

Library of Congress Control Number: 2019912948

Special Thanks to: My wife, my parents and everyone who helped encourage me and my journey through minimally invasive surgery. In no particular order David F, Matthew M, Red, Carlos Z, Richard D, and Trent R.

for Sebastian and Addison.

Foreword

In the most Socratic method possible, I would like to acknowledge the crude and barbaric way this book will read in only a few decades, when our surgical technology will allow such amazing techniques as to render this text akin to a maintenance manual for a Roman chariot.

Q: What is this book?

A: This is an informally written textbook succinctly describing a single surgical technique and how to safely and efficiently perform that technique. It includes patient selection and suggestions for other courses of action for patients who are not candidates.

Q: Who is this book written for?

A: Gynecologic Surgeons of all skill levels. For novices, it will give you the strong opinions of one bossy surgeon to question and challenge. For more experienced surgeons it gives a remarkably candid insight into what one of your colleagues (or competitors,) is truly thinking. This gives you the benefit of either:

1) Reaffirming your own beliefs regarding hysterectomy, and receiving a feeling of pleasure for knowing that great minds think alike, or;

2) Challenging your beliefs with the concepts that I present in this book, and possibly growing your expertise.

Either way, you gain something.

Q: Do you claim that this is the most minimally invasive hysterectomy we can perform in 2019?

A: No, you could still do a completely vaginal hysterectomy, and I recommend doing so in appropriate patients. Also, some authors have used unusual or custom instruments to push the limits a little further, but this is the only described technique using regular commercial equipment that is widely available and inexpensive.

Q: What do you mean by "informally written" textbook?

A: It is meant to be read in the interest of learning the technique and asking yourself if the principles call into question your own surgical decisions and the reasoning behind them. It is also fairly extensively referenced, like most textbooks. It is informal in that there are essentially no tables or graphs, and I write in the first person. Also I say "fuck" a lot.

Q: Would you like feedback?

A: Very much so! Email me at: greg@marchandinstitute.org. Later editions, if produced, will most likely be composed of corrections and updates to the technique, based on input from other surgeons.

Q: Is there somewhere I can watch an example of this surgery being performed?

A: Click this link for a video: https://marchandinstitute.org/singleportvideo

Q: Why did you write this book?

A: Although journal articles (especially in video format) are a great way to share research information, I felt this technique was a little more complex than a single article could encompass. I thought a short, concise book would be the best format to share the technique, as well as to invite feedback from other surgeons. I also thought a "this is what I'm thinking" book would be valuable and comforting to many of my colleagues.

Table of Contents

Chapter 1

Did You Really Just Say You Don't Care Where the Ureter Is?

"I really don't care, in fact I wish him well, 'cause I'll be laughing my head off when he's burning in hell."

-Weird Al Yankovic "Amish Paradise"

When asked about the importance of ureteral dissection at time of hysterectomy, many authors advocate the identification of the ureter, almost without exception. This is both impractical and unnecessary. Dr. Cohen, in her 2019 synopsis of laparoscopic hysterectomy, strongly recommends the same.[1]

This is a waste of time in almost every case. Clearly, ureteral injury needs to be avoided, but entering the retroperitoneum in order to identify the ureter should be a rare occurrence in the career of any gynecologist, outside of the gynecologic-oncologist, and the entry into the retroperitoneum simply for the purpose of stating "I saw it," should be deemed unconscionably reckless.

Instead of identifying the ureter to proudly state that "thou hast seen it," I suggest a new way of looking at the situation: a man from the future arrives and asks if you would prefer a nuclear bomb to blow up in your home or on the surface of Jupiter. Do you need to check Jupiter to be sure your family isn't there? Do you need to call your daughter to be sure she isn't vacationing on Jupiter this week? No, because your family simply cannot be on Jupiter.

There is no way for them to get there, thus this technique. We don't care where the ureter is, because the ureter is not where we are operating. The technique described herein digs into the uterine serosa, and from some aspects may be seen as encouraging other complication from this technique, including the existence of residual uterine serosa that could lead to future fibroid formation, or even sarcoma. What this technique does not allow for, if performed faithfully, is the invasion into the abdomen organs outside of the uterus. Where others have said "see the ureter and cut where it is not," I say, simply, "cut only where the ureter cannot be."

So why am I so scared of retroperitoneal dissection? It's the numbers.[2] Is there any harm in diving into the retroperitoneum to seek out the ureter and find its course? Probably not if you only do it once. Probably not if you do it even twice. Think about how many hysterectomies you're going to perform during your career. For the average gynecologist, it will be in the range of 2,000. For an ultra-high-volume surgeon, it could be multiples of that. If you think that every time you enter the retroperitoneum your surgical skills and the good Lord will save you from a shit-storm injury that requires other specialties to fix, you are sadly mistaken.

Therefore, I humbly present this technique I have developed. Take it from me; when the good Lord decides to shit in your corn flakes, he shall do so, and he shall do so with such force and magnitude that you will regret your course of action for quite some time.

This technique involves an unabashed dissection directly into the uterus. For each bite you take in the initial pedicle dissection, you need to grasp the broad ligament and all adjacent structures and push into the uterus before cutting and burning. For this, I recommend a bipolar electrical cautery device, preferably one that contains a sharp blade for cutting following the cauterization.

At the time of this writing, Covidien's Ligasure™ seems to be the best instrument for this purpose, although I would strongly recommend their 5mm blunt instrument, as their 5mm "Maryland"™ Instrument unfortunately was mistakenly designed with sharp plastic points, and an extremely non-intuitive system of initiating the bipolar energy. The Maryland device requires the surgeon to completely compress the device with the fullest amount of force to activate the energy - there is no other way. This is very unfortunate for two reasons. First, the ultra-sharp plastic points often perform "unintended" dissection into planes that don't need dissection in order to complete this procedure. For this procedure, in essence, the goal is to take all of the pedicles, from fallopian tubes to entering the vagina, with all-encompassing bites of bipolar energy. Each bite pulls together both leaves of the broad ligament, permanently sealing them together in perfect hemostasis, while pushing ever medial, leaving behind a sealed broad ligament, a removed uterus, and excellent hemostasis. Leaving the broad ligament unsealed invariably leads to bleeding, which leads to more lateral application of energy, and that leads to the necessity of cautery adjacent to the ureters. To prevent the last step of this cascade, we need to prevent the first. To do this, we need a strong 5mm bipolar device, and it needs to seal the leaves of the broad ligament as we progress through the procedure.

This seems like a good time to bring up Megatron. Megatron, of course, refers to Da Vinci's™ latest example of whatever robot they are pushing. Video game control of laparoscopy seems seductive, especially in the circumstance of a single-port procedure. However, I warn you - do not be fooled. Megatron is not minimally invasive and arguably may not be laparoscopy.

It has been said that the only true hand-assisted laparoscopy is when you require someone to perform manual masturbation on you in order to obtain the calmness and confidence to perform the procedure - everything else is just a laparotomy.

The same is true with the robotic version of minimally invasive surgery. Centers performing solely single port hysterectomy procedures are reporting herniation rates as high as 23%.[3] Commercial specifications for the Da Vinci SP™ indicate a required incision greater than 2.5cm[4], well outside the size that laparoscopy usually uses. I caution you, this is not minimally invasive surgery.

Three exceptions exist in which robotic usage can be deemed acceptable:

The first is the surgeon who performs only open surgery, who can be taught a simple laparoscopic entry technique, and who can perform a hysterectomy while sitting at the robotic console, unable to grasp the spatial and technical skills required to perform a straight-stick hysterectomy. And, while I would prefer to see this "surgeon" refer his surgical caseload to a more experienced surgeon, it is not unacceptable for him to be taken under the wing of a surgical product representative to learn and master robotic hysterectomy. This is preferable to him or her continuing mostly open hysterectomies.

The second is the reproductive endocrinologist, or any practitioner taking on his caseload. Women desiring pregnancy often require extensive and time-consuming myomectomies, which can benefit greatly from the usage of a robotic surgical platform. Dissecting into the uterine myometrium in order to remove a fibroid and sew up the ensuing incision can be a tricky process using straight stick laparoscopy, and one cannot be faulted for employing the services of a robotic platform for this purpose.[5]

The last exemption from deserved ridicule for robotic usage comes from those practicing gynecologic oncology. Several of my colleagues have stated that the double-articulating arms of the robotic devices provide excellent control for the very articulate dissection of lymph nodes in the area of the large retroperitoneal vessels, most notably the aorta.[6,7]

As I am not a practitioner of these arts,I will take them at their word. For all others, I strongly consider the robotic approach to be both an unnecessary expense (which is forgivable) and an unnecessary extension of operative time (which is *not*.)

References:

1) Cohen, Sara - "Laparoscopic Hysterectomy" UpToDate. Published: 14 Jan 2019, accessed 12 Jul 2019. Wolters Kluwer 2019.
2) Donohue JP, Rowland RG. "Complications of retroperitoneal lymph node dissection." J Urol. 1981 Mar;125(3):338-40.
3) Single-port laparoscopy in gynecologic oncology: seven years of experience at a single institution Moulton, Laura et al. American Journal of Obstetrics & Gynecology, Volume 217, Issue 5, 610.e1 - 610.e8
4) Intuitive Surgical, Corporate Webpage. Retrieved on August 8th 2019, from https://www.intuitive.com/en-us/products-and-services/da-vinci/systems/sp
5) Uterine Myomectomy: Comparing Robot-Assisted, Laparoscopic and Open Techniques Blanton, E. et al. Journal of Minimally Invasive Gynecology, Volume 21, Issue 6, S93
6) Seamon LG, Cohn DE, Valmadre S, et al. Robotic hysterectomy and lymphadenectomy for endometrial cancer: technical aspects and details of success-the Ohio State University method. J Robot Surg 2008; 2:71.
7) Vergote I, Pouseele B, Van Gorp T, et al. Robotic retroperitoneal lower para-aortic lymphadenectomy in cervical carcinoma: first report on the technique used in 5 patients. Acta Obstet Gynecol Scand 2008; 87:783.Vergote I, Pouseele B, Van Gorp T, et al. Robotic retroperitoneal lower para-aortic lymphadenectomy in cervical carcinoma: first report on the technique used in 5 patients. Acta Obstet Gynecol Scand 2008; 87:783.

Chapter 2

Surgical Preparation and Selection of Appropriate Candidates

"If you choose not to decide you still have made a choice.

-Rush "Tom Sawyer"

Success in any procedure is going to revolve around preparation which, for patient benefit, is preparing to perform a hysterectomy one of three ways: laparoscopic single port, laparoscopic multiport, or open laparotomy. Therefore, one can expect a serious and responsible surgeon to have a surgical card with a lot of instruments followed by the words "Hold - Do Not Open."

The patient should be prepped in the dorsal lithotomy position and, if possible, the arms should be tucked. Individual consideration should be given for each obese patient. If a patient is so obese as to not allow the tucking of the arms at the side, then consideration should be given for lateral sleds, if possible, to aid in the appropriate placement of the patient. I would argue against arms extended outward in all but the most obese of patients, secondary to the difficulty for the surgeon to access the appropriate anatomy. If you are in the circumstance where the patient is so obese that arms cannot be tucked, even with the use of, or because of the unavailability of lateral arm sleds, extra-special precautions must be taken.

Laparoscopy usually does not require or amend itself to taping or manipulation of the panus, but in the case where the patient is markedly obese, you will need to look at your operating field not only as an environment in which to perform the laparoscopic procedure, but also as a possible obstacle, should you need to quickly change to an open procedure.

Many of the taping and suspension devices utilized to perform laparoscopy can become time-consuming dangers when immediate laparotomy becomes necessary.

I will try to simplify the discussion as much as possible, with the understanding that every case must be customized based on the obesity of the patient as well as the equipment available in the particular operating room.

At a minimum, in the operating room cutting into an unprepped, or clearly contaminated patient, is unacceptable. Therefore, every laparoscopy must be planned as if immediate conversion to laparotomy is imminent. In some cases of morbidly obese patients or cases of deficient operating room supplies, entering the patient initially laparoscopically in the supine position, after having prepped and draped the patient for laparotomy if necessary, and then proceeding to dorsal lithotomy after pneumoperitoneum is obtained and observing that the intra-abdominal anatomy is amenable to laparoscopic hysetrectomy, is both reasonable and recommended by this author. Any other setup leads to a time delay when converting from the laparoscopic to the open approach, and this could be life-threatening for the patient, especially if the reason for conversion is uncontrolled hemorrhage.

This seems like the ideal time to discuss entry into the obese patient. I hold the very strong belief that, in almost all cases, the best entry into the abdominal cavity is through a natural umbilicus. I state "natural" because a neo-umbilicus, most commonly created by the plastic surgery practitioners, presents with a plethora of problems unique to its own genesis.

Thus, in patients with a neo-umbilicus, individual consideration must be given to the patient's surgical history as well as personal consideration of acceptable cosmesis. (After all, the patient has already had plastic surgery on the abdomen at least once.) Based on this, in all cases of a neo-umbilicus, consideration of a left-upper-quadrant, or "walker point" entry is always reasonable. This is not to say that this is always required. Many neo-umbilicus procedures do not penetrate into the abdomen, and therefore in many cases intra-abdominal adhesions are not suspected. When in doubt, there is no substitute for obtaining previous operative reports.

Moving back to the "run-of-the-mill" obese patient, there is no higher level of safety or more preferred approach than the bottom of the umbilicus. As you push your finger to the bottom of the umbilicus of the anesthetized patient, you are literally holding your finger directly against the patient's fascia. This is true 100% of the time. With the exception of the case where you cannot reach the bottom of the umbilicus, either because of scar tissue, no umbilicus exists, or you simply don't have a long enough finger, identification of this plane should be considered the gold standard approach in all obese patients. One pearl that can be of use in the case of an extremely deep umbilicus is the use of a towel clamp.

Please do not mistake that I would suggest the use of a towel clamp to grasp the patient's fat and lift cephalad, as has been performed by many a well-meaning but disgustingly barbaric laparoscopic surgeon.

Rather, I suggest the towel-clamp because of its rounded head which, when plunged to the bottom of an obese patient's natural umbilicus, will often give a spectacular view of the bottom of the umbilicus, which will then enable you to make an incision with an 11 blade scalpel and subsequently enter with a Veress needle.

This technique, however, should be reserved for the most obese of obese patients. The majority of obese patients have umbilici that can be manipulated manually to reveal the bottom and, upon revealing, a one centimeter incision should be made. You should feel the incision with your finger as the Veress needle "pops" though, as your finger is directly up against the fascia. I would then recommend performing standard Veress needle testing.

Veress needle testing includes attaching a syringe to the Veress needle which is then used, in no particular order, to inject saline, attempt to withdraw fluid from the abdominal cavity, and then demonstrate that fluid will fall through needle into the abdominal cavity when held plumb. If held perfectly plumb, when the lumen of the needle is filled with fluid the tendency of the fluid is to fall into the abdominal cavity, not to remain stagnant or to be pushed outward, secondary to the low pressure in the abdomen.

Conceivably, if your Veress needle is embedded in solid tissue (such as the uterus), fluid could not be injected. Alternatively, in an inappropriate hollow location, such as the bowels, bladder or vasculature, feculent, bloody or urinous fluid may be drawn back. Lastly, the “drop” test of fluid falling in the abdominal cavity is to guard against a pre or post peritoneal entry and, conceivably in the hands of a diligent and experienced surgeon, guard against the unwanted insufflation of the preperitoneal or retroperitoneal spaces. Clearly, insufflation of either of these areas would confuse planes and make effective laparoscopy difficult or impossible.

I have seen many insufflation devices at work and must claim complete ignorance as to their internal workings or function. To be completely honest, I have no idea whether some or all systems are controlled by an internal computer or if it is a “pump until you reach 15mm then stop” system, as simple as the thermostat in my home.

Nevertheless, my stupidity in regard to the function of these machines has not, as in the case of most fools, prevented me from forming a strong opinion. In the topic of insufflation machines I see far better performance stemming from those machines labeled Pneumosure™ and an inferior ability to correctly function on those labeled Highflow 40L™. I have limited, subjective data to support these observations.[8]

So why a Veress needle in the first place? Why not direct entry or Hasson? The answer is deep consideration.

All three entry techniques rely on a single, final step where one penetrates into the unknown layer. The difference with a Veress needle entry is that, in the absence of the true "double skewering" through bowel lumen, the Veress needle entry ***should*** allow the surgeon to know that he has penetrated somewhere he shouldn't have, i.e. the return of feculent fluid or frank blood should clue the surgeon as to what error has occurred. In the case of a bowel injury, a second attempt at laparoscopy can be made through a second site at this point and conceivable the small, usually 9 gauge, Veress needle injury can be repaired without conversion to laparotomy.

In the case of a Hasson or direct entry, this injury will likely need laparotomy and colectomy.[9] In the case of injury to major vasculature, a Veress needle's small caliber will prevent rapid blood loss, giving the surgeon time to convert the setting to a large laparotomy and mend the vessel. An injury to a large vessel from a trocar, even a 5mm trocar, or directly from a Hasson entry, will result in exsanguination in seconds, likely before any surgeon can achieve a laparotomy size-worthy for operative exploration. In medical parlance, we call this a "dire consequence."

As for selection of the appropriate candidate, there are very few characteristics that I would say rule out the possibility of a laparoscopic hysterectomy.[10] Clearly, one excluding factor could be size of the uterus. As many of you know, I have previously used a power morcellator to remove seven pounds of uterus in an 8 hour Guinness World Record™ setting hysterectomy.[11] While this was an interesting surgery, I would not have performed this feat were the surgery planned today. This is not to say that either the FDA black box warning,[12] or the considerable naysayers have at all scared me into believing that leiomyosarcoma occurs with any considerable frequency more than other cancers, or that power morcellation considerably worsens the outcome.[13] Patients who suffer from leiomyosarcoma have an average life span in the range of fifteen months by any data,[14] and the massive number of life threatening complications that have been avoided over the years secondary to morcellation- based techniques avoiding laparotomy is incalculably more valuable.

The real reason, however, that I would not use a laparoscopic power morcellator if I performed the procedure today is the incredible ease and speed at which vaginal morcellation can be performed. Vaginal morcellation is an incredibly valuable, under-taught skill which can enable almost any gynecologic surgeon to remove large masses vaginally. I would highly recommend mastery of vaginal morcellation to all gynecologic surgeons. For those that have this skill, size of uterus is not, in itself, a limiting factor.[15]

While size may not be a limiting factor, features of any individual uterus very well may. **A uterus that will not move when pushed with a vaginal ultrasound probe is trouble.** A uterus that seems to extend to the pelvic sidewall in each direction may make for a difficult hysterectomy. A uterus that is close to spherical in shape will make access to the paracervical pedicles extremely difficult, no matter where trocars are placed. Patients with extensive surgical histories will have scar tissue that will certainly limit surgical access. If that scar tissue has obliterated the posterior cul-de-sac, it can be even more difficult to perform the procedure.

Of all of these, my only true unbeatable enemy is the frozen pelvis. For any that don't know, a frozen pelvis is a state of adhesive disease so advanced that no single significant cavity within the abdomen can be insufflated, and thus, there is really nowhere to begin working from with regards to laparoscopy. This will be evident upon entry into the abdominal cavity, where even with the tip of the trocar clearly in the abdominal cavity, no cavity opens.

In a case like this, there is no other recourse than to slowly withdraw your entry and examine carefully for bowel or vascular injury, and consider whether a second attempt can be made. Traditionally, a left upper quadrant entry can be attempted in a case such as this, after adequate decompression of the stomach using a nasogastric tube. From my experiences, this is usually just a confirmation to prove what you already know from your original entry - laparoscopic technique is impossible in this scenario. I would encourage less experienced surgeons to attempt the left upper quadrant entry in your first few encounters, in order to be sure what you thought you saw in the umbilicus was the whole story. There is the possibility of expanding omental adhesions in the area of the umbilicus, which can rarely give the convincing illusion of a frozen pelvis in an abdomen otherwise amenable to laparoscopic surgery. A true frozen pelvis however, even in the hands of an expert surgeon, forces the hysterectomy to the vaginal or open approach.

Counseling any patient with any of the above features should differ from your "norm," with explanations given as to why the particular circumstance of the procedure raises the possibility to conversion. As discussed in the next chapter, however, with the exception of patients that refuse a particular modality for personal preference, the decision of abandoning laparoscopic single port for laparoscopic multiport, or abandoning multiport for laparotomy, should only be made at the time of surgery, and specifically at the time of first visualization of the abdominal cavity through the umbilical port.

References:

8) Nepple, K. G., Kallogjeri, D., & Bhayani, S. B. (2013). Benchtop evaluation of pressure barrier insufflator and standard insufflator systems. Surgical endoscopy, 27(1), 333-338.
9) Compeau, C., McLeod, N. T., & Ternamian, A. (2011). Laparoscopic entry: a review of Canadian general surgical practice. Canadian Journal of Surgery, 54(5), 315.
10) Marchand, G; Demir, R (September 5, 2012). "Irrelevance of Traditional De-Selectors for Minimally Invasive Hysterectomy". Journal of the Society of LaparoEndoscopic Surgeons, Presented at the 2012 Conference, Boston, MA, doi: 10.13140/RG.2.2.11424.89601.
11) Marchand, G; Demir, R (Oct–Dec 2010). "Safe Laparoscopic Removal of a 3200 Gram Fibroid Uterus". Journal of the Society of Laparoendoscopic Surgeons. 14 (4): 600–602. doi:10.4293/108680810X12924466008169. PMC 3083059 . PMID 21605532.
12) US Food and Drug Administration, November 2014, " Immediately in Effect Guidance Document: Product Labeling for Laparoscopic Power Morcellators: Guidance for Industry and Food and Drug Administration Staff" www.fda.gov
13) Demir, RH "Incidence of Uterine Sarcoma in 1432 Consecutive Minimally Invasive Hysterectomies," Journal of Minimally Invasive Gynecology, Volume 22, Issue 6, S35
14) Wang, Z., Shi, N., Naing, A., Janku, F., Subbiah, V., Araujo, D. M., ... & Ramirez, P. T. (2016). Survival of patients with metastatic leiomyosarcoma: the MD Anderson Clinical Center

for targeted therapy experience. Cancer medicine, 5(12), 3437-3444.

15) Magos, A., Bournas, N., Sinha, R., Richardson, R. E., & O'Connor, H. (1996). Vaginal hysterectomy for the large uterus. BJOG: An International Journal of Obstetrics & Gynaecology, 103(3), 246-251.

Chapter 3

Preoperative Counseling

"No one who respects the law and likes to eat sausage should ever watch either being made."

-Benjamin Franklin

To explain the prefacing quote, the line is meant to explain or draw homage to those surgeons who make it a point of discussing every possible complication of a surgery simply for the purpose of attempting to talk the patient out of the surgery, or to attempt to send the patient somewhere else. I'm not ashamed to say that I have seen this strategy undertaken much more often by practitioners who are on salary as opposed to those paid as a percentage of their productivity. While there is certainly nothing dishonorable about doing whatever you can to get out of a surgery that you do not feel comfortable doing, there is something wrong with overstating the risks of an otherwise routine procedure to a patient who needs it. I think it is reasonable to broadly go over possible complications, but an in-depth discussion of what it is like to have a bowel movement through the colostomy is not appropriate for standard hysterectomy. “Injury to the bowels, bladder, urine tubes, or blood vessels” will suffice.

My experiences observing colleagues explain surgical procedures to patients in the preoperative area have been disturbing, to say the least. For the purposes of this text, I’m going to limit the discussion to appropriate counseling for a hysterectomy, as the premise of this text is that you are trying to offer your patient the most minimally invasive hysterectomy possible. My several world records demonstrate that you have indeed come to the right place to achieve this endeavor. But how we might offer preoperative counseling, in simple terms, is a deeper question.

I believe the best counseling comes from statistic-based analysis. If you open half of the hysterectomies that you perform, your patient deserves to know this, (although the same could be said with regard to your state medical board.) My suggestion is to come up with a statistical analysis by looking at your past data. Decimal points are not important, but commonly experienced complications should be described as common.

One particular pearl is the subset of patients that fear a urinary catheter more than they fear death itself. A urinary catheter is a painful thing without question, but different patients have different capacities to tolerate this. If a woman has multiple cesarean sections, and is deathly afraid of the presence of a postoperative urinary catheter for any extended period of time, then this should be discussed extensively preoperatively. An extensive discussion should be had with the patient regarding the nature of scar tissue following cesarean sections and the necessary dissection to bring the bladder off of the uterus. It should also be discussed that this dissection may result in a cystotomy, and that the successfulness of this dissection will absolutely be based minimally upon the skill of the surgeon and mostly on the already-present scar tissue from the patient's prior cesarean sections. If she is so absolutely and pathological afraid of an indwelling catheter, although it pains me to even type this out - this patient may be better served with a laparotomy.

In the end, unique to this described technique, you must inform the patient that this surgery will be accomplished one of three ways: laparoscopic single port, laparoscopic multi-port, or an open Pfannenstiel laparotomy.

I don't think it is necessary to discuss with the patients who are not candidates for laparoscopic hysterectomy, but clearly not every patient is. A patient with a 50cm uterus does not need this discussion. Barring these very unusual cases, ***the ideal time to decide the proper route for the hysterectomy will be at time of entry into the abdominal cavity, usually through the umbilicus, and decisions for method of completion of the surgery should be reserved for that time alone.*** You should provide your patient with your best estimates based on your skill, previous accomplishments, and of course your assessment of the patient's individual risk factors. These will certainly include, but not be limited to, including their weight, uterine size, previous abdominal surgeries, and any previous accounts of the quantity of intra-abdominal adhesions.

One additional aspect of preoperative preparation which should not be overlooked is the necessity to be aware of the anesthesia available. I am not an across-the-board proponent of all of the ERAS (Enhanced Recovery After Surgery) protocol, or other protocols that depend on multiple factors in order to theoretically improve postoperative recovery. From my experiences at multiple institutions, restricting eating and drinking or failing to do so has essentially no bearing on the patient's recovery, and whatever minor hunger pangs occur from the patient missing breakfast before surgery, they have no bearing on recovery whatsoever. This is not to say I'm a stickler for an 8 hour fast (quite the contrary, there is probably no harm to throwing the old NPO rules out the window), I believe that there is no real benefit with regards to postoperative recovery.

As for the preoperative carbohydrate drinks, I also think the data behind this practice is useless. There is no flavor of Kool-Aid™ that will make your patient's wounds heal faster, and shame on you if you thought there was.

Finally, while early feeding and carbohydrate rich solutions in the intraoperative period are utter bullshit, I am convinced that ***combined spinal and general anesthesia is not***. I am uncertain about the reasons for this and I am uncertain that anyone truly understands the reasons why this anesthesia is superior, but it simply is true.[16] When I converted my ultra high-volume hysterectomy service from general anesthesia to a combined spinal general service, we went from patients who had a 20% chance of requesting a second hospital day postoperatively to patients that routinely had to be warned to avoid sexual activity immediately following surgery. The results were *that* good.

As a surgeon, it is beyond my scope to understand the physiology of why this occurs or perhaps I am just not smart enough. Whatever the reason, combined general anesthesia with epidural or spinal anesthesia is a requirement for any minimally invasive hysterectomy, and if anesthesia that can provide these services is not available, I would recommend delaying the procedure until such services *are* available.

References:

16) Ghodki, P. S., Sardesai, S. P., & Naphade, R. W. (2014). Combined spinal and general anesthesia is better than general anesthesia alone for laparoscopic hysterectomy. Saudi journal of anaesthesia, 8(4), 498.

17) Suryavanshi, V. S., Sahu, A., & Harde, M. (2016). Efficacy of combined epidural general anesthesia for attenuating haemodynamic responses in gynaecological laparoscopic surgery. International Journal of Contemporary Medical Research, 3, 1354-8.

Chapter 4

Talking to the Difficult Anesthesiologist

"I would not trust that doctor to take care of my DNR goldfish. Even if I really thought that Mr. Wiggles had lived a good life and it was truly his time."

- Marchand

Fuck it. They never listen. If they won't do spinal-general, cancel the case and make sure next time you've got it set up with someone who will do it. Apologize profusely to the patient.

Chapter 5

Selection of Vaginal Manipulator

"Vaginal Manipulator Means More to me than just a nickname in High School"

-Anonymous

In a difficult single-port hysterectomy, choice of vaginal manipulator will absolutely make or break the procedure. Conversion to multiple-port or open hysterectomy will be much more likely when limitations on uterine manipulation exist. Nonetheless, not every community hospital can be convinced to purchase the most expensive manipulator on the market, and not every hysterectomy can be performed in your favorite tertiary center. As a result, sometimes you just have to make do.

Let's start off with some eliminations: a Sponge-Stick, RUMI™, Cohen, Hulka and a McCartney Tube™ without the manipulating lumen are not compatible with this technique.

Although I appreciate greatly down-sizing surgical costs, you are better off channeling your inner MacGyver to create a vaginal manipulator using a uterine sound and a snapped apart laparoscopic trocar than you would be using a sponge-stick to expose the fornices to create a colpotomy. It is just too low-tech.

The RUMI™, or at least the initial design, has a handle which creates an angle that is not amenable to hysterectomy in humans. Although later models may have solved this problem, I'm still not sure how that original angle was created. You just can't manipulate the uterus at all with a straight rod. I am left dumbfounded.

Also, a McCartney Tube™ devoid of its manipulating center is equally useless, although it could be utilized in the case of an extremely small uterus. For those of you not familiar with the McCartney Tube™, it is essentially a long rubber-like cylinder inserted into the vagina with an open edge to make your colpotomy against. In other words, it's like an empty Cambell's soup can made of rubber. This provides a great view of the surface for your circumferential colpotomy but essentially no manipulation of the uterine body. In all but the lightest of wombs, this is incompatible with a single-port laparoscopic technique.

I will now move to the gold standard, the McCarus-Volker "Fornisee™." This product is amazing and has a price tag equally as daunting. The Fornisee™ device contains an adjustable uterine manipulating rod, at a perfect angle, and the rod itself is solid steel. It can move any amount of tissue without bending. It also has an adjustable tip that turns horizontally to lock into place in the uterus. The burning surface is perfectly angled and is made of a hard, plastic-like substance that does not melt or change shape even when burned directly with 50 watt coagulating monopolar current. Finally, that ring that you want to make your colpotomy on, you know that final ring you trace around to complete the hysterectomy? Have you ever "missed it?" You know what I mean, the tissue was too thick, you were a little caudad or a little cephalad and just not on the ring? Well let me tell you this, **this ring lights up**.

Yes - I shit thee not!

This ring actually has a light making the exact level of the colpotomy easily visible throughout the entire procedure. You read that correctly, the entire procedure, because this ring is lit. (By the way it is not hot and will not burn any tissues.) So, operating with this device is very much like having the wind at your back.

Not every hospital is going to have this device, so some good substitutes would be the Colpotomizer™, Uterine ElevatOR PRO™, V-Care™, and the RUMI II™ (with the arch). Any of these will be able to manipulate the uterus to expose every aspect, which is what you're going to need if you've only got one port to work with, because a traction port just isn't available. Just remember that seeing the ring in the initial surveillance of the abdomen can be very important, because you can only judge how much work it will really take to complete the single-port hysterectomy if you can see when the work will be finished.

Chapter 6

Choice of a Power Device

"Then, when you have found the shrubbery, you must cut down the mightiest tree in the forest... with... a herring!

The Knights Who say Ni, Monty Python and the Holy Grail

Many of us remember fondly the good old days of residency when hysterectomy meant a large incision and a lot of clamping, tying and cutting. Those days are long gone.

The entire laparoscopic hysterectomy, whether performed with a robot, single-port or multiport, is dependent on the use of a very powerful power device in order to cut the pedicles. As with the previous sections I'm going to start off with devices that I think are not suitable.

First and foremost I would eliminate the harmonic scalpel. Vibration energy is a very novel and interesting tool for surgery, unfortunately I have found no use for it in gynecologic minimally invasive surgery. When a colleague tells me that they are about to perform a surgery using a harmonic scalpel I ask them how many units of blood they have typed and crossed.

Attractive as it may be, an Endo GIA™ device is also off-limits secondary to the presence of staples. Although there is nothing inherently wrong with using a surgical clip to stop bleeding on a laparoscopic field, metal objects in the vagina or that can come into contact with the area adjacent to the vagina with mechanical motion should be avoided at all costs.

A novel technique is to use bipolar energy on a small device and then use a second instrument to actually cut the pedicle after desiccating the tissue using the bipolar energy. This technique has been demonstrated using miniature laparoscopic devices and can be done through extremely small 3mm laparoscopic ports.[18,19] The obvious limitation of this technique is that the small nature of the ports make them extremely flimsy, and they are useless as this technique requires strong power instruments that push into the uterus in order to avoid spaces which might conceivably contain the ureter.

Acceptable devices will include all devices that utilize bipolar energy. I'm going to mention the Enseal™, the Thunderbeat™, the Ligasure™ and the Tripolar™ devices. All of these are acceptable, convenient devices that can be used to accomplish this technique. Of these, I would recommend the Ligasure™ and particularly the five millimeter blunt Ligasure™ device. I am aware that the company no longer actively markets this product and, instead, they're actively marketing a new device which is named after the state containing Baltimore.

The Maryland device has several significant flaws. First, unlike the soft edges of the blunt device, the Maryland device instead has sharp plastic tips which tend to get you into planes that you don't really want to be in. For example, when using it you may often find yourself inside one of the leaves of the broad ligament instead of sealing the two leaves together en masse as this technique recommends.

But that's not the biggest problem with the device. The biggest problem is that the activator button on the device for the bipolar energy is hidden at the foot of the lever that closes the jaws. Therefore the energy activates only when you pull the handles all the way down. Even if 100% of the energy of pulling down the handles isn't transmitted to the jaws, you just don't want to be pussyfooting around the ligaments and uncertain that you have a good grasp of them because you are afraid of activating the bipolar device, as invariably occurs. This leads to a surgical technique that is devoid of the finesse necessary to repeatedly slide the bipolar device snugly against the uterus to perform the safest hysterectomy possible. Therefore, I avoid the Maryland Ligasure™ if it all possible. I would like to mention that the 10 millimeter blunt Ligasure Atlas™ is a great device[20], however it would be incompatible with our single-port technique secondary to the large size. The Atlas™ remains my device of choice when cutting through larger tissues laparoscopically. It is particularly useful on very large fibroid pedicles using the technique of multiple burns as the jaws slowly close more and more with each successive burn.[21]

References:

18) Fanfani, F., Fagotti, A., Gagliardi, M. L., Monterossi, G., Rossitto, C., Costantini, B., ... & Scambia, G. (2013). Minilaparoscopic versus single-port total hysterectomy: a randomized trial. Journal of minimally invasive gynecology, 20(2), 192-197.
19) Uccella, S., Cromi, A., Casarin, J., Bogani, G., Serati, M., Gisone, B., ... & Ghezzi, F. (2015). Minilaparoscopic versus standard laparoscopic hysterectomy for uteri≥ 16 weeks of gestation: surgical outcomes, postoperative quality of life, and cosmesis. Journal of Laparoendoscopic & Advanced Surgical Techniques, 25(5), 386-391.
20) Demirturk, F., Aytan, H., & Caliskan, A. C. (2007). Comparison of the use of electrothermal bipolar vessel sealer with harmonic scalpel in total laparoscopic hysterectomy. Journal of Obstetrics and Gynaecology Research, 33(3), 341-345.
21) Takeda, A., & Nakamura, H. (2016). Torsion of a subserosal myoma managed by gasless laparoendoscopic single-site myomectomy with in-bag manual extraction. Case reports in obstetrics and gynecology, 2016.

Chapter 7

Entry into the Abdomen - aka "The Whole Enchilada"

"Gee Wilikers, it must be obvious day on camp stupid."

- Master Shake, Aqua Teen Hunger Force

I will begin with the assumption that every high-volume, minimally-invasive-preferring surgeon has very strong feelings about his or her entry into the abdominal cavity. By the time you've completed your 1000th laparoscopy, I am quite certain that you will be set in your ways and it will be difficult to convince you that my way is correct and that your way is wrong. Let me attempt this, anyway.

Hasson umbilical entry, or so called "open laparoscopy" is a nonsensical technique that is barely worth mentioning in this text. It neither improves the safety of entry into the abdominal cavity, the cosmesis of that entry, nor is it more minimally invasive than any other technique. It is fundamentally flawed from a minimally-invasive surgery perspective and yields no advantages.[22,23] The concept that cutting down through the layers of the abdominal wall (none of which provide any difficulty for laparoscopic entry), will help you with the final layer is ridiculous. All of the danger of the final step of entry is present, regardless of how you got to the final layer. The "open laparoscopy" entry simply leaves the surgeon with a larger final incision and the same necessary entry beyond the peritoneum into the abdominal cavity, with a greater chance of enterotomy or other injury than the below mentioned techniques.

Optical trocar systems that allow you to visualize your entry are not necessarily bad, but provide no actual advantage.[24,25] Unlike the flawed Hasson technique that results in a larger incision on the skin and in the final entry to the abdominal cavity, optic systems merely fool the surgeon into believing that visualizing the entry gives them any power to control the final entry into the abdomen. This is not the case. The final layer is the final layer, whether you can see it or not.

Direct entry into the abdominal cavity with a blunt trocar is an excellent technique, however counter traction on the abdominal wall can be difficult to maintain, especially in patients with either too much or too little body fat. Direct entry with a sharp trocar is not advised as the non-insufflated abdomen will yield many obstacles and a large bladed trocar will very likely create complications. You're also left with the problem of how to hold countertraction with the abdominal wall. This leads to the unfortunate and quite brutal action I have seen many surgeons take of grasping the abdominal wall with towel clamps. The clearly correct entry is to first use a Veress needle to insufflate.[26]

This gives the surgeon the unique advantage of being able to first inject and then withdraw saline into the abdominal cavity, which gives extremely valuable information about the location of the tip of the needle. The Veress needle is generally less than 2 mm in diameter, so in the unfortunate circumstance that you have put your needle into an object you did not intend to, it is extremely likely that this will not be a catastrophic error. An incidental enterotomy that is created with a Veress needle can be easily recognized before you unintentionally place a large trocar into the same loop of bowel. Assuming that you can then choose a different entry site and obtain a pneumoperitoneum, this small 2 millimeter injury can easily be oversewn from the laparoscopic approach with minimal difficulty. Injuries to the vasculature with a 2 mm needle are also clearly going to be less dangerous. I hope that I never see any item in my operating room penetrate the aorta, but I would certainly prefer a small needle hole than the entry of any size trocar should that day come that the good Lord calls my number.[27]

So, where to place your umbilical incision? No matter how skilled of a surgeon you are, there is always a benefit to using the advantages you are given. Feel the bottom of anyone's umbilicus, yes, even yours if you want to, feel it right now and you will see that it interfaces directly with the patient's fascia.

No matter how much fat there is, if you've truly found the bottom of a natural umbilicus, you are at the fascia. This anatomical rule always holds true - as long as you can find the bottom of someone's belly button! This law will work for any degree of morbid obesity. Therefore, if you can get to the bottom of the patient's belly button, you can get right up against a patient's fascia. If you can get your Veress needle right up against the bottom of the patient's belly button, then you have your Veress Needle right up against the fascia. All you need to do then is make a small skin incision and pop the needle through.

As discussed above, using this technique does not free you from any possibility of complications. If that very tiny 2 mm area of the fascia that you are entering into has densely adhered intestines on the other side, then your number is up. Fortunately, since it's just a 2mm hole you'll more than likely be able to detect your error and correct it, whereas entry by some other means cannot escape serious complications easily.

As an interesting and ironic mention, an ideal instrument for visualizing the bottom of a patient's umbilicus and for making your incision with an 11 blade scalpel at the bottom of an obese patient's umbilicus is a towel clamp. In this case, we are not talking about using the towel clamp in the barbaric way many surgeons do, grasping the tissue and pulling up. Rather, we leave the towel clamp closed and use an 11 blade scalpel through the end of the clamp. In this way, the towel clamp is actually acting as a 320 degree retractor for the walls of the patient's umbilicus. Surgeons that choose to master this technique become masters of entry for laparoscopy in even the most obese of patients.

If you want to use this technique in a patient with a neo-umbilicus, you may be justified in doing so. The umbilicus that the plastic surgeon created may very well interface very close to the fascia but, unlike those created by God, there is no guarantee that the fascia will be there. Still, in my opinion, it is an excellent way to enter the patient from a cosmesis perspective in an area that will be extremely unlikely to have a wound infection in the postoperative period.[28,29]

Following insufflation with the Veress needle, you can then proceed to place an 11 millimeter blunt trocar through the umbilicus and examine the abdominal cavity with a laparoscope. This brings us to the "Moment of Truth" that will be the subject of Chapter 8 as we make important decisions regarding the approach.

So, let’s say you've done everything right, made a small incision at the very bottom of the umbilicus, you inserted your Veress needle right through the fascia, you've injected saline, received no fluid back and a positive drop test into the abdominal cavity all confirms good placement. All this was done correctly, and yet you still can't insufflate. The insufflator keeps flashing between "15" and "obstruction." What is wrong and what do you do next?

Ideal entry into the abdominal cavity with the Veress needle would have been tilting the Veress needle approximately 30 degrees toward the patient's feet, generally directly in the midline. I would withdraw the needle at this point and attempt another Veress needle entry except this time also slanting the needle 30 degrees to the left or the right.

I would be prejudiced about which direction by any prior scars on the patient’s abdomen and, in the case that no scars exist, I would probably go toward the patient's right because I'm standing on the left side of the table and it seems a more fluid motion. In the obese patient, your Veress needle angle is generally straight down into the abdominal cavity to maximize the chance of entering the abdominal cavity, and I generally never use an extended- or bariatric-size Veress needle.

In the case of an obese patient, I would change my angle for the second entry to be more toward the patient's feet, perhaps at an inflection of 15 degrees caudad. I would again try to insufflate the abdominal cavity and, if unsuccessful a second time, switch to a direct entry through the incision that we have created in the umbilicus with a 5mm blunt trocar. Of course, I would never proceed with insufflation if any of the various needle injection and withdrawal tests showed concerning results. Obviously, concerning results would be the inability to inject saline into the abdominal cavity, which would indicate the tip of the needle being in a solid object, the withdrawal of frank blood or feculent material, or a negative drop test.

Clearly, each of these scenarios needs to be dealt with and some of these scenarios require immediate laparotomy. To continue with my protocol, if I am unable to enter the abdominal cavity through the umbilicus, I would change to a left upper quadrant point and attempt to insufflate the abdomen in that area without making an incision, after asking anesthesia to deflate the stomach via nasogastric tube.

If I am able to insufflate from the left upper quadrant, I would then return to the umbilicus and again attempt blunt entry into the umbilicus with a slightly more caudad angle using a five millimeter trocar. My rationale would be that the peritoneum is now pushed firmly against the fascia and upward secondary to the insufflation, so entry is much more likely to be successful at this time.

If I'm not able to insufflate using only the Veress needle from the left upper quadrant, I would then abandon the possibility of performing the intended single-port technique and instead enter the left upper quadrant directly using a small incision and a 5 mm blunt trocar. If I'm still unable to insufflate and visualize the abdominal cavity, I would give consideration to possible insufflation from the vaginal approach, using the posterior cul-de-sac, before abandoning laparoscopy altogether.

The high success rate of the left upper quadrant entry justifies its usage when umbilical entry fails,[30,31] although the obvious downside is that if your left upper quadrant entry fails you will then need to inspect for injuries in the left upper quadrant with a laparotomy which would normally be quite low in the pelvis. This inspection from a Pfannenstiel can be very challenging, and you may need to be satisfied with the absence of obvious bleeding from this area in difficult patients.

References:

22) Lam, A., Kaufman, Y., Khong, S. Y., Liew, A., Ford, S., & Condous, G. (2009). Dealing with complications in laparoscopy. Best Practice & Research Clinical Obstetrics & Gynaecology, 23(5), 631-646.
23) Johnston, K., Rosen, D., Cario, G., Chou, D., Carlton, M., Cooper, M., & Reid, G. (2007). Major complications arising from 1265 operative laparoscopic cases: a prospective review from a single center. Journal of minimally invasive gynecology, 14(3), 339-344.
24) Sharp, H. T., Dodson, M. K., Draper, M. L., Watts, D. A., Doucette, R. C., & Hurd, W. W. (2002). Complications associated with optical-access laparoscopic trocars. Obstetrics & Gynecology, 99(4), 553-555.
25) McKernan, J. B., & Finley, C. R. (2002). Experience with optical trocar in performing laparoscopic procedures. Surgical Laparoscopy Endoscopy & Percutaneous Techniques, 12(2), 96-99.
26) Vilos, G. A., & Vilos, A. G. (2003). Safe laparoscopic entry guided by Veress needle CO2 insufflation pressure. The Journal of the American Association of Gynecologic Laparoscopists, 10(3), 415-420.
27) Azevedo, J. L. M. C., Azevedo, O. C., Miyahira, S. A., Miguel, G. P. S., Becker, O. M., Hypólito, O. H. M., ... & Freire, D. (2009). Injuries caused by Veress needle insertion for creation of pneumoperitoneum: a systematic literature review. Surgical endoscopy, 23(7), 1428-1432.

28) Neri, V., Fersini, A., Ambrosi, A., Tartaglia, N., & Valentino, T. P. (2008). Umbilical port-site complications in laparoscopic cholecystectomy: role of topical antibiotic therapy. JSLS: Journal of the Society of Laparoendoscopic Surgeons, 12(2), 126.
29) Hamzaoglu, I., Baca, B., Böler, D. E., Polat, E., & Özer, Y. (2004). Is umbilical flora responsible for wound infection after laparoscopic surgery?. Surgical Laparoscopy Endoscopy & Percutaneous Techniques, 14(5), 263-267.
30) Patsner, B. (1999). Laparoscopy using the left upper quadrant approach. The Journal of the American Association of Gynecologic Laparoscopists, 6(3), 323-325.
31) McDanald, D. M., Levine, R. L., & Pasic, R. (2005). Left upper quadrant entry during gynecologic laparoscopy. Surgical Laparoscopy Endoscopy & Percutaneous Techniques, 15(6), 325-327.

Chapter 8

The Moment of Truth

"In any moment of decision, the best thing you can do is the right thing, the next best thing is the wrong thing, and the worst thing you can do is nothing."

- Theodore Roosevelt

I refer to this point in the surgery as "The Moment of Truth" because this is the point where the surgeon should correctly ascertain the best way to complete the procedure. There are a number of factors that are going to tell you if this procedure can be completed by single-port laparoscopy, multi-port laparoscopy, or, in rare cases, by laparotomy. You're going to need to look at all of these factors and consider the probability of success for each.

It will also be important to consider what your individual strengths are as a surgeon. In addition to thoroughly surveying the abdominal cavity from the laparoscopic approach, there are three quick maneuvers that will give you a little more information as to how much trouble you are in. First, light the vaginal ring and gently move it to see where exactly the plane is. Next, gently move the uterus with the uterine manipulator and see how much mobility the uterus has. Lastly, gently challenge the anterior adhesions with the laparoscope, if necessary. All of these techniques will be described below.

First of all, it is critical for you to think about what it is that you are removing, meaning what really needs to be removed, and what the patient would tolerate being left behind if it meant a more minimally invasive surgery. Hopefully you've discussed with the patient all the different possible scenarios, and you'll feel as if you have a good grasp of what the patient would want. If you can complete the hysterectomy laparoscopically but you're not sure you can remove that ovary, would the patient really want you to remove that ovary? Does she have a history of ovarian cancer in her family? Is she having this surgery in the first place for pain on that side? Clearly, it is critical to consider all possible scenarios and counsel the patient appropriately prior to putting them to sleep. It would be quite tragic if you felt you had to cut the patient open for an ovary that you later learned they would have preferred left behind. The applications of this train of thought should extend to all manner of laparoscopic procedures in gynecology, not just this hysterectomy technique.

Next, let's look at what adhesions are in the way. What do you really need to go through in order to remove the uterus and the other organs we need to take out? Are the adhesions really blocking the path, or can they be pushed to the side? Am I thinking about doing more surgery than I need to? What is inside those adhesions, and am I sure I know that? Can they be safely cut or is there a chance they contain bowel or other organs I don't want to damage? A quick move for gaining a little more insight may be to place your 5 mm laparoscope a little deeper into the abdominal cavity so that you can visualize the abdominal walls a centimeter or two away from the front scope. Next, ignore the wall as you quickly do a 360 degree panoramic rotation around the abdomen and see what adhesions are still in place after you have made the full circle. Clearly, you do *not* want to put too much pressure on the laparoscope if adhesions have your scope stuck in place, at least not at this point in the procedure.

Next, try to visualize the ring of your vaginal manipulator. If you are using the Fournisee™, light it up and see where the ring is. All other manipulators will require some wiggling at this point to see how much of the outline of the ring you can visualize. Can you visualize it at all before you've gotten it any pedicles? Is the posterior cul-de-sac completely obliterated, or can you see a safe plane at the bottom lip of the vaginal manipulator ring? Can you manipulate the uterus to see more of it? Look at the interface of the bladder with the ring. Can you see where the bladder stops? If you're not sure, you may want to fill the bladder by retro-filling with saline using your Foley catheter. I can't tell you how many times this technique has saved me from creating a bladder flap that wasn't even necessary, in a bladder that was enough out of the way to just complete the hysterectomy without dissection. The bottom line for your dissection is that if you can get to the ring safely you can finish the procedure.

Lastly, let's look at the size of the uterus. Can it be removed vaginally without morcellation? If I do need vaginal morcellation, am I skilled enough at vaginal morcellation to complete this? If I poke at the uterus does it seem soft? Has the patient had a course of luprolide™ that has made it rock-solid? There is little point in performing a complete hysterectomy laparoscopically if you then cannot remove the uterus without laparotomy, but there is also a great benefit in improving your vaginal morcellation techniques, even at the expense of operative time.

Now, consider whether you can complete this hysterectomy with a single port technique. If you cannot, can you complete it with a multi-port technique? Also, if you feel so inclined, there is nothing wrong at this point with concluding laparoscopy and performing a vaginal hysterectomy as you were trained. As you become more accustomed to this technique, the quick assessments of the abdomen, uterus, ring and adhesions become part of the first steps of your procedure. You may even wish to take down a few easy first pedicles in order to test your assumption. We have all had the experience of being surprised at how easily some hysterectomies go that we originally thought to be quite difficult, and how quickly "gimme" cases can turn into hysterectomies that we have needed to open or came very close to needing to do so. I am of the mindset that a true frozen pelvis, as well as a completely obliterated posterior cul-de-sac, will always require a laparotomy. I am generally able to avoid laparotomy in most patients, but always keep in mind that the "good old bikini cut" is far preferable to any patient than a bladder, ureteral, or bowel injury. Remaining chapters will focus on assuming you have gone forward with the single-port laparoscopic approach as described.

I did not mention the type of trocar preferred for this entry, as any type of 11 millimeter blunt trocar can be used. I am quite fond of the Ethicon™ trocar as well as the Covidien™ trocar. The Applied Medical Trocar™ is a less desirable product as the plastic point of the trocar does not make sense for entry at the abdominal cavity and does not include any type of plastic "blade". Any blunt trocar, including a reusable trocar, would be acceptable for the purposes of this technique.

If you have surveyed the abdomen and are going forward with a single port hysterectomy, the next step is to remove your blunt trocar and insert the introducer Ring of the Olympus Tri-Port™ device into the abdominal cavity. Depending on how thick the abdominal wall is, the ring may be placed through the footprint of your 11 mm trocar Port manually, or you can use the introducer that comes with the Olympus Tri-Port™ device to inject the base ring into the abdomen. After you have removed your 11 mm blunt trocar, depending on the type of trocar utilized, your incision will either be almost exactly the same diameter as the introducer on the tripod, or slightly smaller. Either way, it is not important because all that you need to do at this point in the surgery is to match up the introducer to the incision and inject the contents, which contain the plastic base ring and some of the plastic sheet of the Olympus Tri-Port™ device, into the abdominal cavity. It is a rare complication for the ring to lodge between the peritoneum and the fascia, and if it does it is fairly easy to withdraw the ring using the collapsible strap and then deploy the ring a second time. If too much time passes and the abdomen begins to desufflate, you may need to replace the 11 mm port to re-insufflate the abdominal cavity and make another attempt at placing the Olympus Tri-Port™ device.

From this point, once you or the introducer has placed the ring in the abdominal cavity, you will firmly pull up on the sleeve, trim the sleeve and install the triport device in the normal manner. The only exception, of course, is that the device is now installed through an 11 millimeter incision created by a blunt laparoscopic trocar, instead of the recommended size which ranges from 1.5 to 3 cm.[32,33]

So what is our thought process behind using only an 11mm incision and creating that incision using an 11 mm blunt trocar as opposed to creating the incision directly with a scalpel or using a bladed trocar? This is a difficult question. I'm not going to dive into a debate going over all of the literature of laparoscopic entry and the different trocar port sizes, and the respective necessity to close each individual port size, whether it be bladed, blunt or "step-up," with suture in order to avoid port-site hernia. There has been a lot of data released lately about single-port procedures performed with a robot and an abysmally high complication rate **(5.5% omg!)** with regards to umbilical hernias following oncologic procedures including hysterectomy.[34,35]

Unlike the common medical journal article, I have a more effective tool to make my point with. The most important and easily accepted piece of information is the one that builds on information the surgeon already knows to be true. There are many ultra-high-volume, minimally invasive laparoscopic surgeons in the United States.[36] Most of these are very comfortable using at 11 mm blunt trocar port, and the data is controversial about whether this port needs to be closed.[37,38]

Personally, I have performed over 3,000 laparoscopic surgeries using the port and have never had an umbilical port site hernia. Although it is my practice to attempt to close the fascia from the abdominal approach (not laparoscopically) I would assume that at least one of these closures would have failed over the years if the closure was really necessary, especially in light of my less-than-stringent rules for closure of the 11mm bluntly created incision, which will be further discussed in Chapter 15. Therefore, in my mind, at 11mm and blunt we are always safe.

For ultra-high-volume surgeons, it's not just the avoidance of the port site hernia, it's also our comfort with the recovery from incisions this size. Ultra-high-volume minimally invasive surgeons are very, *very* used to performing 10 or more surgeries per week, and having little or no complications. Patients go home with holes no bigger than 11 mm and it's essentially unheard of for these incisions to become infected. Even in uncontrolled diabetics and patients with immunosuppressive disorders, these tiny incisions getting any type of infection postoperatively is essentially unheard of.[39] I believe this argument makes the most sense to high-volume surgeons, since this procedure is geared to those very same ultra-high-volume laparoscopic surgeons.

Therefore, I humbly present this technique which will allow us to perform a complete laparoscopic hysterectomy, the most common major surgery we perform, through the very same incision that we have become so accustomed to for our other "bread and butter" laparoscopic surgeries. I will admit that, initially, I was suspicious about the reproducibility as well as the success of this procedure, but now that I have performed dozens of these procedures I am convinced that this technique is a very optimal way to perform a hysterectomy with minimal recovery. Further, when this procedure is used with a combination of spinal and general anesthesia, the result is an incredible, ultra-minimally invasive technique which literally removes the majority of postoperative pain and suffering from a major surgery that many women need.

This brings us to the main impetus for my technique, as minimally-invasive surgeons that do extremely high volumes of surgery, hysterectomy seems to be the one surgery that we commonly lose sleep over. Following hysterectomy, we commonly worry about the ureters, lose sleep over possible complications, and are awakened in fear at 3:00 AM by nurses asking questions or needing orders on patients that are staying overnight. My overall goal with this technique is to reduce that fear and to bring this very common procedure firmly back into our toolbox of "everyday" procedures we can perform on an outpatient basis, without any fear of serious complications.

Now, if you've installed the Triport™ in the 11mm incision, congratulations! You have now completed the preoperative setup for the Single Port Advanced Laparoscopic Hysterectomy.

Let's move on to the good stuff!

References:

32) Müller, E. M., Cavazzola, L. T., Grossi, J. V. M., Mariano, M. B., Morales, C., & Brun, M. (2010). Training for laparoendoscopic single-site surgery (LESS). International Journal of Surgery, 8(1), 64-68.

33) "Single Site (LESS) Appendectomy | Olympus America | Medical". https://www.medical.olympusamerica.com/procedure/single-site-less-appendectomy. Retrieved 2019-07-14.

34) Moulton, L. J., Jernigan, A. M., & Michener, C. M. (2017). Postoperative outcomes after single-port laparoscopic removal of adnexal masses in patients referred to gynecologic oncology at a large academic center. Journal of minimally invasive gynecology, 24(7), 1136-1144.

35) "Single-Port Laparoscopic Surgery for Gynecologic Cancers is Safe and Effective, but What About Hernia Risk?". https://consultqd.clevelandclinic.org/single-port-laparoscopic-

36) surgery-for-gynecologic-cancers-is-safe-and-effective-but-what-about-hernia-risk/. Dated 2017-12-07. Retrieved 2019-07-13

37) Lim, P. C., Crane, J. T., English, E. J., Farnam, R. W., Garza, D. M., Winter, M. L., & Rozeboom, J. L. (2016). Multicenter analysis comparing robotic, open, laparoscopic, and vaginal hysterectomies performed by high-volume surgeons for benign indications. International Journal of Gynecology & Obstetrics, 133(3), 359-364.

38) Swank, H. A., Mulder, I. M., La Chapelle, C. F., Reitsma, J. B., Lange, J. F., & Bemelman, W. A.

(2012). Systematic review of trocar-site hernia. British Journal of Surgery, 99(3), 315-323.

39) Lago, J., Serralta, D., García, A., Martín, J., Sanz, M., Pérez, M. D., & Turégano, F. (2011). Randomized prospective trial on the occurrence of laparoscopic trocar site hernias. Journal of Laparoendoscopic & Advanced Surgical Techniques, 21(9), 775-779.

40) Yim, G. W., Jung, Y. W., Paek, J., Lee, S. H., Kwon, H. Y., Nam, E. J., ... & Kim, S. W. (2010). Transumbilical single-port access versus conventional total laparoscopic hysterectomy: surgical outcomes. American journal of obstetrics and gynecology, 203(1), 26-e1.

Chapter 9

Choose Your Weapons

"A man can never have too much wine, too many books, or too much ammunition."

- Rudyard Kipling

So now you've got your flexible Triport™ installed in your 11 mm umbilical incision and it's time to select your weapons. First, let's look at the possibilities. An 11 mm incision, as a perfect circle, provides approximately 95 square millimeters of space. Each 5 mm instrument you place through the incision takes roughly 20 square millimeters of space and, because these are solid instruments, not liquid, you have to allow for room around adjacent objects as they will not change their shape. One advantage, however, is that the incision itself can change shape. The diameter of the incision should stay the same (no stretching!) whether the incision is pulled to a perfect circle or stretched more front to back or side to side. Therefore an oval configuration or more of a triangular configuration will usually be the shape the incision is held to, all while keeping the same diameter. As a result, even though 3 circles each having a 5 mm diameter cannot fit inside of one circle with an 11 mm diameter, you can pull the diameter into a more triangular shape to accommodate all instruments without the need for extending the diameter.

At this point, I'll give my recommended initial configuration. I would recommend a 5 mm, 30 degree laparoscope, unless you do have an articulating scope available. There are several excellent articulating laparoscopes, and if you have one available I would recommend using it. Always take every advantage you have at your disposal. This technique, however, was designed with the idea that only a 30 degree 5 mm classical laparoscope will be available, in order to make the technique as widely reproducible as possible. With the exception of the $250 single port device that can be purchased online,[40] I will wager that all of the instruments required to perform this procedure are found in 99% of hospitals with operating rooms or surgery centers in the United States at this very second.

As for your other starting instruments, I recommend starting with the 5 mm blunt Covidien Ligasure™ device, (although as stated any 5mm bipolar energy device will suffice). I also recommend having a 5 mm non-traumatic (wavy) grasper available for any part of the procedure that requires it. This can be easily threaded between the two existing 5mm instruments for difficult portions of the case, and removed for easier portions to reduce instrument "clanging."

There are several different devices which a surgeon may wish to have available to complete this procedure. The majority of this surgery is completed with the surgeon's dominant hand on the bipolar device and the nondominant hand on the vaginal manipulator. This should then change, upon reaching the vaginal cuff, for a monopolar Bovie™ type device in the dominant hand. The third instrument that can be used either by the surgeon or by the assistant will vary according to the clinical scenario. I would recommend having a 5 mm laparoscopic tenaculum (single tooth), a 5 mm Endo Kittner™, and several different types of nontraumatic graspers available in case they are needed. A suction irrigator should also be available, although my goal, and hopefully yours as well, will be to complete the procedure without enough blood loss to justify the use of the suction irrigator.

References:

41) ESuture.Com - Olympus Triport Device - https://www.esutures.com/product/0-in-date/69-olympus/101-miscellaneous/46243827-olympus-triport-15-laparoscopic-instrument-port-kit-WA58015T. Retrieved 2019-07-12

Chapter 10

Initial Pedicles and Where is the Ring?

"Before You Die You See The Ring"

-Rachel Keller, The Ring (2002)

As stated, the majority of the procedure should be performed with the main surgeon having one hand on the Ligasure™ and the other hand firmly on the uterine manipulator.

This can be somewhat counter-intuitive for laparoscopic surgeons who are used to performing procedures using two hands, and manipulating an instrument in each (i.e. grasper and power instrument.) In this case, the surgeon manipulates the uterus against his or her bipolar ligating device, and later against the monopolar cautery, and we perform almost the entire procedure from this perspective. The assistant will be used to expertly position the camera, especially in executing the advanced technique of positioning the camera in a more lateral than natural perspective in order to best use the 30 degree offset to best visualize the operating field.

Again, I would prefer a Fornisee™ lighted uterine manipulator if available, secondary the multiple advantages it entails, however any vaginal manipulator with a ring that can be visualized can be used. Skilled positioning of the camera is critical to the success of the technique, therefore the assistants must become experts at placing the camera in a "counterintuitively" lateral position in order to use the 30 degrees offset to the surgeon's best advantage.

This is *literally* the opposite goal of direct visualization during robotic surgery, and can take quite a bit of practice to master. Care must be taken as to whether the camera is best positioned above or below the operating instrument based on the position of the uterus and the body habitus. If every movement of the operating instrument moves the camera as well, although this may be a necessary annoyance for difficult parts of the procedure, this is not the ideal circumstance for the entire procedure. Dissection should progress from this perspective and should then go forward, taking the major pedicles of the uterus, including the fallopian tubes, round ligament, both leaves of the broad ligament, the cardinal ligament and the uterine artery. I recommend combining as many of these structures in as few bites as possible. I would recommend taking the bites through the ligaments as aggressively as possible, and with each bite the jaws of the power instrument should be snug against the uterus. Using the recommended bipolar devices will result in the sealing of the anterior and posterior lips of the leaves of the broad ligament, which will result in excellent hemostasis. As reported by many authors, I recommend pushing cephalad with your vaginal manipulator so that you are actually performing the circumferential colpotomy on the Ring of the vaginal manipulator cephalad to the utero-sacral ligaments.[41] Leaving the utero-sacral ligaments intact and attached to the vagina is a critical step of this hysterectomy and may have serious implications for preventing prolapse of organs later in the patient's life[42] (although some authors dispute this theory[43]).

A concept central to this entire hysterectomy is that these bites should be taken directly against the uterus if not within the uterus itself. Clearly this technique is not amenable to any type of cancer surgery where the intention is to remove surrounding tissues to prevent the spread of cancer. I also agree with the recommendation of other authors with the tenet that the removal of the Fallopian tubes is not appropriate at the time of initial hysterectomy, and that the Fallopian tubes should be removed later, after the uterus has been removed vaginally and even possibly until after the vaginal cuff has been sewn.[44] Doing so limits danger to the ureters and removes unnecessary interference in visualization. Bites should be taken on each side of the uterus until all ligaments are ligated and divided to the level of the circumferential colpotomy. Multiple burning of individual pedicles may be necessary at times, and as long as the plane of dissection is kept snug against the uterus, no fear of lateral energy spreading is needed, regardless of device.

The next task that must be accomplished is the creation of a bladder flap and the movement of the bladder out of the operating field. Clearly, this task will be best accomplished with good visualization of the interface between the bladder and the uterus. As a manner of habit, I generally reduce all possible pedicles on each side of the uterus before turning attention to the bladder flap. Actual creation of the bladder flap is probably best made using the bipolar energy device after the uterine manipulator is used to push the uterus as laterally as possible to the patient's right side. This usually involves shifting the power device slightly to the right to come across the top of the isthmic portion of the uterus in order to create a plane in the uterine serosa. Radical pressure to move the uterus laterally from the vaginal manipulator can usually produce close to a 90 degree angle for this dissection.

Alternatively, this dissection can also be performed with an endoscopic extension on a Bovie™ device, although even with coagulating energy this will not be as hemostatic as the bipolar. From here, it should be relatively easy to push down the bladder using either the bipolar device or a second instrument such as a wavy grasper or Endo Kittner™ device. If there is any doubt that the entire bladder has been successfully removed from the operating field, consideration should be given for immediate backfilling of the bladder with saline through the Foley catheter in order to be sure the cephalad edge of the bladder is out of the operating field. Repeated filling, drainage and dissection may be required in complex cases. In cases of dissection where it becomes very difficult to see exactly where the bladder plane is, extreme precaution should be given to allow the possibility of leaving uterine serosa on bladder tissue, as opposed to the extremely unfortunate event of a cystotomy. As discussed in previous chapters, some patients fear the indwelling presence of a Foley catheter more than the actual pain or risk of the surgery itself. Following the division of all pedicles and the creation of a bladder flap, circumferential colpotomy should be the last step in the hysterectomy from an abdominal approach.

For this procedure, the recommended tool is a Bovie™ cautery device with a laparoscopic hook extension attachment. Preferably 35 watts of coagulating current should be used, as cutting current is unnecessarily deficient in hemostasis, and the vaginal vault has an excellent blood supply that one need not fear interrupting. I would also highly recommend a handheld Bovie™ device, with controls in the surgeon's hand as opposed to a foot pedal. Stepping on foot pedals can be cumbersome and also adds an additional element of danger to the surgery, especially if unintentional activation of the power device occurs. Clearly, manipulation of the 30° laparoscope will be necessary in order to visualize the anterior and posterior portions of the uterus in order to form the circumferential colpotomy.

There are several techniques that you must learn in order to successfully and quickly perform the circumferential colpotomy. First, the anatomical location of the bladder and the nature of the anterior abdominal wall mean that it is much safer to have your cautery bounce off into the anterior aspect of the abdomen than the posterior aspect, and therefore it will be preferable to perform your colpotomy from a posterior to anterior approach. The best tool for this will be the laparoscopic extended hook cautery, and I would again suggest this be attached to a hand-held monopolar Bovie™ device, not with a cumbersome foot pedal. You should begin the colpotomy after all pedicles have been dissected and the bladder has been pushed well out of the operating field.

Please note that, although in this technique I only recommend closing the vaginal cuff and not specifically closing the parietal peritoneum, if your goal will be to modify my technique to close the parietal peritoneum as well, then you're going to have to push the bladder even farther out of the operating field in order to leave yourself enough room so as to sew the two leaves of the peritoneum together. If you were following the techniques in this book to the letter and not closing the peritoneum then you simply need to move the bladder out of the area of the colpotomy to complete the procedure.

Once you are sure that all pedicles are hemostatic, you've pushed the bladder out of the way of the impending colpotomy, and you have denuded the tissue in the paracervical area to expose the outline of the manipulator ring all the way around, you can begin the colpotomy. I recommend beginning the colpotomy by grasping the posterior vagina with the endo-hook either directly against or, in some configurations, placed into the groove of the vaginal ring of the manipulator. I recommend starting on whichever side you feel will be the easier side, and starting your colpotomy from about 5 to 15 degrees on the contralateral side of the absolute bottom of the manipulator ring.

Thus, you will almost immediately be crossing the midline as you perform your colpotomy. I recommend using coagulating current as there is no danger of stripping this area of the anatomy of its robust blood supply. My common setting is 35 watts of coagulating current. You should then complete the first half, (or 55-65%) of your colpotomy and then switch to the opposite side, ending at approximately the absolute top of the vaginal ring. If the tissue has been properly denuded and all vessels ligated prior to the colpotomy, you will often find that no further dissection is necessary and that you can cleanly make the colpotomy in one pass. Ideally you would then move to the other side and finish the remaining 140-160 degrees of the colpotomy from that side. Although the manipulator ring, even when coupled with a rod-like uterine body manipulator, does not have the ability to “swivel” the vagina very much against the ring, the small amount of movement that can be performed can be extremely useful and, in difficult cases, can allow you to visualize the start of your contralateral colpotomy so that you can continue the incision all the way around in one motion. Mastery of these twisting movements of the manipulator is critical for fast, efficient, repeatable colpotomy. It's also critical that the bladder edge is pushed out of the operating field prior to attempting to complete the colpotomy. Dissection in the area of the utero-vesico fascia is described above.

The techniques for performing circumferential colpotomy depend heavily on the ability to sustain a pneumoperitoneum at time of colpotomy. As I have done in previous aspects of this surgery, I will rate for you the methods for obtaining pneumoperitoneum from worst to best. The absolute worst is the attempt of packing the vagina with moist laparotomy sponges in order to achieve pneumoperitoneum. In my opinion this has the same effect as “wishing really hard.”

A slightly more effective approach will be to pack those wet sponges inside sterile surgical gloves and then pack those in the vagina. This also usually fails, especially if a vaginal manipulator is constantly dislodging them. The superior practice will be the use of pre-manufactured pneumo-occluder balloons. These balloons can be useful for maintaining pneumoperitoneum, however I would strongly recommend filling those balloons with saline instead of air, and know ahead of time exactly how far you can get away with insufflating them without the balloon bursting. Manufacturers are notorious for suggesting that you under inflate their balloons below maximum efficacy so that you will never have a balloon rupture inside a patient.

Lastly, if you want the best, as so often is preferred in life, you have to pay for it. The previously described Fournisee™ has a rubber pneumo-occlusion ring that, once placed in the vagina, essentially never fails, regardless of the amount of manipulation.

I recommend turning off the insufflation while leaving the Tri-Port™ in place as you move the vaginal perspective. Please be mindful of escaping pneumoperitoneum vaginally, especially if you are not wearing eye protection!

References:

42) Koh, C. H. (1998). A new technique and system for simplifying total laparoscopic hysterectomy. The Journal of the American Association of Gynecologic Laparoscopists, 5(2), 187-192.
43) Rahman H, Trehan N (2017) 'Adenomyosis': The Enigma. Adv Laparoscopy 1(1):29-33.
44) Schaffer, J. I., Wai, C. Y., & Boreham, M. K. (2005). Etiology of pelvic organ prolapse. Clinical obstetrics and gynecology, 48(3), 639-647.
45) Tormena, R. A., Ribeiro, S. C., Maciel, G. A., & Baracat, E. C. (2015). Single-port laparoscopic hysterectomy: preliminary results. Revista da Associação Médica Brasileira, 61(5), 446-451.

Chapter 11

Time to Remove the Uterus (Without using the "M" Word)

"The alternative to morcellation is to remove the uterus intact through an abdominal incision (abdominal hysterectomy)."

-ACOG

Back when I completed my formal surgical training, and dinosaurs roamed the Earth, laparoscopic hysterectomy was an extreme minority. As a result, whenever we just completed all the pedicles on a vaginal hysterectomy and found the uterus was simply too large to remove vaginally, we used a technique we called "bivalving the uterus." This method allowed us to remove the mass of uterus vaginally. This is, of course, referring to making a bisecting incision in the uterus, most commonly cervix-to-fundus, which changes the maximum diameter of the uterus so that it can fit out the vaginal orifice.[45] After performing this procedure multiple times, it just simply became second nature and that by repeatedly bivalving or repeatedly making incisions into the uterus to express a smaller diameter of uterine body, essentially any size uterus could be removed through the vagina. Uteri as large as 3,000 grams have been removed by this technique.

Although conceivably any size uterus could be "bivalved" in such a manner that it never becomes more than one "piece," similar to spiral-cutting a single orange into a 6 foot length of peel and triangles, in reality no one did that in my training and no one would ***ever*** do that. We performed the "bivalving," removed some tissue, repositioned, got a little more, and so on, until all the uterus was out, likely in quite a few pieces. What we were really doing was manual vaginal morcellation. As the average gynecologist's skill-set had moved away from vaginal hysterectomy and toward laparoscopic hysterectomy in the last decade, the art of removing large masses vaginally is a skill in decline.

Fast forward a few decades and we have "morcellation," a term once associated with the most innovative advancements in laparoscopic surgery, which has now become an extremely controversial word that brings fear to the heart of any hospital administrator. There are many reasons that abdominal power morcellation fell out of favor in the last 10 years.[46] Some of this has to do with injudicious patient selection, and many practitioners have used abdominal power morcellation on patients that were not appropriate candidates. ***Uteri that can be removed vaginally always should be, and always should have been.***

Another reason had to do with the absence of data to definitely disprove the benefit of supracervical hysterectomy,[47,48] and since posterior colpotomy with a cervix in place is a more rare skill,[49] this also may have resulted in more abdominal morcellation than necessary. Whatever the reason, this culminated with a 2014 FDA Black Box warning about using power morcellators and the possibility of spreading leiomyosarcoma.[12]

The majority of the cases of spreading leiomyosarcoma were a direct result of poor patient selection. In other words, surgeons that easily could have removed uteri vaginally did not, and continued the laparoscopy or robotic assisted surgery just because they could. But this is not to say that abdominal power morcellation does not have its place. Some tissues, especially ovarian, can be reliably ruled out as malignant. In other circumstances, patients may simply be too sick with comorbidities to reliably recover from a midline laparotomy. Lastly, in some cases, such as a fertility sparing myomectomy, the patient may choose to forgo the large laparotomy once they understand the risks of morcellation, and should be entitled to the less invasive surgery if that risk is understood. Suggesting that power morcellators should be banned is akin to suggesting chemotherapy to a patient that did not have cancer and then complaining that the side effects of the chemotherapy meant that all chemotherapy should be banned.

In honest retrospect, ***there just weren't that many cases where power morcellation was really needed.*** Any skilled gynecologic surgeon will quickly realize that removing masses through a colpotomy, even a posterior colpotomy with a retained uterus, is a faster, easier, safer technique, and it is one that is extremely worthwhile to master.

Vaginal removal of the uterus, regardless of its size, will be the preferred modality for completing this laparoscopic technique. Although most uteri will be able to be removed without "bivalving" (vaginal morcellation), the technique is a critical component of this surgery.

References:

46) Grody, M. H. T. (1989). Vaginal hysterectomy: the large uterus. Journal of Gynecologic Surgery, 5(3), 301-312.
47) Wright, J. D., Chen, L., Burke, W. M., Hou, J. Y., Tergas, A. I., Ananth, C. V., & Hershman, D. L. (2016). Trends in use and outcomes of women undergoing hysterectomy with electric power morcellation. Jama, 316(8), 877-878.
48) Kuppermann, M., Summitt, R. L., Varner, R. E., McNeeley, S. G., Goodman-Gruen, D., Learman, L. A., ... & Showstack, J. (2005). Sexual functioning after total compared with supracervical hysterectomy: a randomized trial. Obstetrics & Gynecology, 105(6), 1309-1318.
49) Milad, M. P., Morrison, K., Sokol, A., Miller, D., & Kirkpatrick, L. (2001). A comparison of laparoscopic supracervical hysterectomy vs laparoscopically assisted vaginal hysterectomy. Surgical endoscopy, 15(3), 286-288.
50) Pillai, R., & Yoong, W. (2010). Posterior colpotomy revisited: a forgotten route for retrieving larger benign ovarian lesions following laparoscopic excision. Archives of gynecology and obstetrics, 281(4), 609-611.

Chapter 12

Meaningful Vaginal Closure

"You don't need closure. You just need to give yourself permission to move on."

–Steve Harvey

Following the removal of the uterus, whether or not there needs to be any manipulation of the uterus to remove it, I'm a firm believer that the best next course of action is to close the vagina from the vaginal perspective. There are several reasons I hold this belief. Initially, there was some data to show that vaginal closures were more successful than abdominal closures and there was a lower rate of vaginal dehiscence.[50,51,52]

Recent data has called into question whether this is true for all levels of surgical experience.[53] Nonetheless, closure from the vaginal approach has several large advantages.

First of all, for the majority of women who had a vaginal delivery, closing the vagina from the vaginal approach is very fast and easy. One simply needs to grasp any aspect of the vaginal cuff that can easily be palpated in a Kocher clamp. From there, a quick running locked suture, preferably with 0 vicryl or larger on a CT needle, is all that is required and can easily be performed through a speculum. In rare cases and more difficult circumstances, assistance with vaginal retractors can be helpful. Following completion of the vaginal suturing, you should immediately test the suture by gently pushing up either with your fingers or a vaginal sponge stick. A successful vaginal closure need not be airtight (although it would be nice), but it should be successful to the point where a sponge stick when inserted in the vaginal approach cannot be visualized in the abdominal cavity at time of returning to laparoscopy. No part of the white sponge should be seen from the abdominal approach.

Some difficult cases may not be able to be closed vaginally and, in this case, multiple authors have published techniques including novel practices such as barbed sutures that do not require tying and closing the peritoneum without closing the vaginal cuff at all.[54,55] In the event that vaginal closure of the vaginal cuff is not possible, I recommend the best closure possible from the abdominal perspective using whichever instruments the surgeon is most comfortable using. If it happens to me, I fall back on my EndoStich™ device with 2.0 PolySorb™ to complete the closure from the laparoscopic perspective. If, after "failing" to close the vaginal cuff from the vaginal perspective, the vaginal cuff cannot be closed abdominally, I recommend closing the peritoneum abdominally and putting in some sutures vaginally as well.

Following closure of the vaginal cuff, I would recommend the surgeon completely change his or her gown and gloves, as removal of the uterus and sewing of the vaginal Vault are going to make it almost impossible to keep the surgical gown sterile. I have seen some surgeons simply change their gloves at this point of the technique, but I think it is most appropriate to completely change the gown and gloves and scrub back into the procedure. At this point the surgeon should resume the abdominal aspect of the procedure and turn the insufflation back on. The abdominal cavity should again be visualized. The vaginal cuff should be visualized by gently pushing a sponge stick in the vagina under direct laparoscopic visualization. This check has two purposes. First, you must be sure that no part of the sponge on the sponge stick in the vagina is visual in the abdominal cavity and, if it is seen, consideration should be given for placing additional stitches from the vaginal perspective. Alternatively, one could place additional sutures from the abdominal perspective if thought feasible. (***Please be sure to remove the sponge stick first to avoid sewing it permanently into the patient's vagina.***) As previously stated above, it is not necessary for the vaginal closure to be airtight, but it is critical that none of the sponge be visualized from the abdominal cavity. A second reason for testing the vaginal vault with the sponge stick, while visualizing laparoscopically, is to be sure that none of the bowels are attached to the suture line.

Generally, an intrusion into the bowels with suture is not a large problem, after all suture (of smaller caliber) is commonly used on the bowels for anastomosis and over-sewing when necessary. Therefore, when invasion into the bowels of the vaginal suture line is detected, further interventions are likely unnecessary. All that is required is to carefully cut the suture from the vaginal perspective and re-suture the vaginal cuff while being careful that the offending bowel is no longer in the operating field. Following inspection of the vaginal cuff, if the surgeon is satisfied with the integrity of the newly sutured vaginal cuff, attention can be turned to the adnexa.

Clearly, discussions regarding retaining or removing the ovaries must be performed as part of reasonable counseling for any hysterectomy. While ovarian preservation will always be a controversial topic outside the scope of this text, it is difficult to imagine any circumstances where any Fallopian tube tissue should be retained at time of hysterectomy. Following the advent of Committee Opinion #620, there is really no excuse for leaving the tubes, barring one possible exception.[56] That exception will be the occasional Fallopian tube that is so deformed that it is clearly plastered on the lateral side wall. In this case, removing this tube could require extensive dissection of the retroperitoneum, and you're probably better off leaving behind some Fallopian tube tissue than to dive into the patient's retroperitoneum in order to make a dissection in close proximity to the ureter.

As the uterus has been removed, the medial aspect of the Fallopian tubes should be fairly easy to identify, in most cases, because of the burns. Removal of the Fallopian tubes on each side should be undertaken separately from removal of the ovaries, in order to minimize the amount of retroperitoneal tissue taken in each bite. A secondary grasper is generally not necessary, as this technique recommends placing only the bipolar energy device behind the Fallopian tube, and the Fallopian tube should be gently pulled medially in the abdominal cavity. You should have the jaws of the bipolar device snug against the Fallopian tube without any unnecessary tissue in the jaws. Multiple bites should be taken in sequence until the Fallopian tube is free from the abdominal side wall.

All of this dissection should take place in the middle of the abdominal cavity, far from the lateral side walls, in order to prevent any unnecessary spread of electricity to structures in the retroperitoneum.

Following removal of the Fallopian tubes, removal of any ovaries that the patient wants removed should occur. The bipolar energy device should be placed behind the ovary and the ovary should be held as medial as possible, prior to activating the Ligasure™ device and cutting the ovarian ligaments. Pressure should be held medially with special care not to tear the ligaments. Pressure should be essentially as much as can be reasonably applied without fear of ripping the infundibular pelvic ligament.

This technique of keeping snug against the ovaries has been criticized by several authors because of its risk of ovarian remnant syndrome.[57] While this risk does exist, the risk of ovarian remnant syndrome and subsequent morbidity is quite small compared to the risk of ureteral injury, which is a devastating complication of hysterectomy. Therefore, I would recommend that only in select cases should surgeons abandon the technique of "snug" removal of the ovaries, perhaps in some chronic pain patients. The rationale is that, while dissection with the bipolar "snug" against the ovary does have the potential of leaving microscopic amounts of ovarian tissue, it is extremely valuable in avoiding injury in the adnexa.

In an abdomen with severe adhesive disease, this precaution becomes doubly important. Following the separation of the ovaries and the Fallopian tubes from the adnexa, they should be removed from the abdominal cavity, either in an endocatch bag or whole if possible. Removal of instruments in the opening of the abdominal Port will generally provide enough room to remove these tissues without any morcellation. "In-bag morcellation" can be utilized when appropriate and necessary to remove larger ovaries. The technique simply refers to exteriorizing the mouth of the bag and using ring forceps to remove pieces of the tissue until the bag can be withdrawn.

Clearly, careful attention must be paid to not damage the bag in any way, as this could cause contents to leak back into the abdominal cavity. I have previously used this technique to remove a very large ovarian tumor and then completed the staging laparoscopically with the assistance of a gynecologic oncologist.[58]

Following the removal of the adnexa, the abdomen and pelvis should again be surveyed,and special attention should be paid to the vaginal cuff. For this technique I recommend placing one unit of powdered coagulant on the vaginal cuff to aid with hemostasis (Arista™ or Surgicel Powder™). I prefer this technique as opposed to closely watching the vaginal cuff while simultaneously decreasing the pressure of the pneumoperitoneum.

I believe the technique of placing a hemostatic agent is generally successful in stopping small areas of bleeding of the vaginal cuff, which will prevent hematoma and subsequent abscesses. One important precaution I will give is to guard against the use of Surgicel™ or any other "sheet" shaped coagulant agents on the vaginal cuff.[59] Patients often present to emergency rooms following hysterectomy, and when a patient presents with one of these objects, invariably containing air, is it extremely likely the emergency room staff will believe that the patient has an abscess.

Following this, it is unfortunately quite common for surgeons who are unfamiliar with the primary surgery to perform a repeat laparoscopy or laparotomy in search of the suspected abscess. Therefore, I would recommend only powdered coagulant agents at time of hysterectomy.

Lastly, we finish our anesthetic efforts by injecting 20 cc's of one half percent marcaine directly into the abdominal cavity, in all patients except those with extremely small body mass index.[60] The thought process behind this injection is that it can be easily soaked in by all pedicles and will help with the post-operative pain. While my evidence for this is largely anecdotal, I will gladly state that no patient has ever woken up from a hysterectomy and said that, while they had no pain in their abdomen or pelvis, they had severe pain from the tiny incisions on their skin. Therefore, with this reported from thousands of my laparoscopy patients, I would not suggest numbing the incisions in the skin but instead suggest using the marcaine in the abdominal cavity where it can do the most good.

References:

51) Kho, R. M., Akl, M. N., Cornella, J. L., Magtibay, P. M., Wechter, M. E., & Magrina, J. F. (2009). Incidence and characteristics of patients with vaginal cuff dehiscence after robotic procedures. Obstetrics & Gynecology, 114(2 Part 1), 231-235.

52) Robinson, B. L., Liao, J. B., Adams, S. F., & Randall, T. C. (2009). Vaginal cuff dehiscence after robotic total laparoscopic hysterectomy. Obstetrics and gynecology, 114(2 Pt 1), 369.

53) Uccella, S., Ceccaroni, M., Cromi, A., Malzoni, M., Berretta, R., De Iaco, P., ... & Ghezzi, F. (2012). Vaginal cuff dehiscence in a series of 12,398 hysterectomies: effect of different types of colpotomy and vaginal closure. Obstetrics & Gynecology, 120(3), 516-523.

54) Uccella, S., Malzoni, M., Cromi, A., Seracchioli, R., Ciravolo, G., Fanfani, F., ... & Corrado, G. (2018). Laparoscopic vs transvaginal cuff closure after total laparoscopic hysterectomy: a randomized trial by the Italian Society of Gynecologic Endoscopy. American journal of obstetrics and gynecology, 218(5), 500-e1.

55) Siedhoff, M. T., Yunker, A. C., & Steege, J. F. (2011). Decreased incidence of vaginal cuff dehiscence after laparoscopic closure with bidirectional barbed suture. Journal of minimally invasive gynecology, 18(2), 218-223.

56) Einarsson, J. I., Cohen, S. L., Gobern, J. M., Sandberg, E. M., Hill-Lydecker, C. I., Wang, K., & Brown, D. N. (2013). Barbed versus standard suture: a randomized trial for laparoscopic vaginal cuff closure. Journal of minimally invasive gynecology, 20(4), 492-498.

57) Committee on Gynecologic Practice. (2015). Committee opinion no. 620: Salpingectomy for ovarian cancer prevention. Obstetrics and gynecology, 125(1), 279.
58) Rana, N., Rotman, C., Hasson, H. M., Redwine, D. B., & Dmowski, W. P. (1996). Ovarian remnant syndrome after laparoscopic hysterectomy and bilateral salpingo-oophorectomy for severe pelvic endometriosis. The Journal of the American Association of Gynecologic Laparoscopists, 3(3), 423-426.
59) Marchand, GJ., Pile, R. Successful complete laparoscopic staging of ovarian cancer in a patient with a 17 cm malignant ovarian tumor. 4th International Conference on Gynecology & Obstetrics. October 04, 2017 Barcelona, Spain.
60) Young, S. T., Paulson, E. K., McCann, R. L., & Baker, M. E. (1993). Appearance of oxidized cellulose (Surgicel) on postoperative CT scans: similarity to postoperative abscess. AJR. American journal of roentgenology, 160(2), 275-277.
61) Marchand, G. J., & Sainz, K. M. (2015, April). Single Port Laparoscopic Hysterectomy through a 12mm incision created by a Bladeless Trocar: A Novel Technique. In BJOG-AN INTERNATIONAL JOURNAL OF OBSTETRICS AND GYNAECOLOGY (Vol. 122, pp. 121-121). 111 RIVER ST, HOBOKEN 07030-5774, NJ USA: WILEY-BLACKWELL.

Chapter 13

The Horrible Way the World will end if you Don't Close the Fascia

"An integral part of any relationship is knowing that you could be killed in your sleep at any time."

- Trent Reznor

So you finished the hysterectomy abdominally, left the multiport device in the umbilicus, and desufflated the abdominal cavity with the port still in place. After this, you've gone to the vaginal approach and closed the vaginal cuff. After closing the vaginal cuff, you placed a sponge stick in the vagina and returned to the abdominal perspective, turned the CO2 back on, and visualized the abdominal cavity. At this point, you have removed any ovaries or fallopian tubes that you needed to, placed some Arista™ on the vaginal vault. Next you pulled the Triport™ and now it is finally time to close the fascia. ***Or is it?***

The debate of whether or not suturing to close the fascia is necessary is a debate that is almost as old as laparoscopy itself. Clearly, umbilical hernia is a disastrous complication of laparoscopy, essentially requiring a second surgery.[61] This surgery, in many cases, is felt by the patient to be more intrusive than the first. Not to mention the fact that a surgeon who *"can't get things right the first time"* will be considered poorly by his colleagues and patients.

Closing the fascia, however, is not without risks itself. Routine fascial closure will invariably increase operative times and, in situations where fascial closure could be more difficult, you must raise the possibility of a complication. The most notable of these complications is bleeding, which could go unnoticed as the fascial incision is closed. This is not to say that incision site bleeding is completely avoided by avoiding fascial closure, as there is the occasional blood vessel held in tamponade by the trocar port and which, upon removal of the trocar port, will bleed. It is just more common to have bleeding with the suturing of fascia at the end of the laparoscopy procedure.[62]

Delving into the data is of very little use in this issue. Multiple authors have argued the necessity to close ports of greater than 12 mm.[63] Multiple others have argued the necessity to close ports created with sharp trocars. Considerably fewer authors have argued closing incisions less than 12 mm, and even fewer authors have argued the necessity to close smaller incisions created by blunt trocars.[64]

In the interest of patient safety, speedy expeditious nature of surgery, and most importantly, reproducibility of this technique, I offer this compromise: ***the college try***.

To clarify, I am not suggesting that closure of the fascia is a trivial item. If anything in the surgery has forced you to expand the size of the umbilical incision, for example, or if you have also used the umbilical incision to remove a mass encapsulated in a bag which stretched the walls, or if an overzealous resident or surgeon-in-training has stretched the umbilical incision using his or her fingers, then without a doubt a true closure of the fascia must take place.

For a true closure of the fascia, I generally recommend any one of the laparoscopic closure systems, the Carter-Thomason™ system being the most famous.[65] In the event that you are using only a single port, a fascial closure technique using S retractors or Army/Navy retractors will be acceptable, as well. However, for the majority of cases performed with this technique, there is likely no reason the fascia needs to be closed, which is why I recommend only closing those which are easily visible. I recommend inspecting the umbilicus, inspecting the subcutaneous tissue and seeing if the fascia is easily noticeable from gentle inspection using only pickups or Addison forceps.

In the event that you are able to visualize both sides of the fascia, by all means grasp those by the tissue planes and close them. My favorite suture for this is 0 Vicryl on a UR 6 needle.

However, in the event that you cannot clearly see the fascia, I do not recommend you begin an intrusive expedition to locate it if you have only used a bluntly created 11mm port. Instead, I recommend simply closing the subcutaneous tissue that you are sure is not within the abdominal cavity with a single interrupted suture. This will help to approximate the size of the fascia and, at least temporarily, will prevent any herniation of bowel contents through this hole. Most importantly, this closure of the subcutaneous tissue will allow you to comfortably place your Dermabond glue into the skin incision without the fear that this glue is going to enter the abdominal cavity where it could be considered quite caustic.

I generally do not recommend a cutaneous suture other than the Dermabond™ glue. It is also recommended that, in order to achieve the best results after placing the subcutaneous suture or fascial suture at the bottom of the umbilicus, you should gently push the umbilicus into the abdomen prior to putting the glue inside of it. This will return the umbilicus to a nice concave shape that, almost invariably, it will heal into permanently. This is both cosmetically pleasing to the patient and provides an excellent "tiny bowl" to pour the Dermabond™ glue into. Following the surgery, most patients find they have a smaller, more concave umbilicus than they previously had, and many patients compliment me on how their umbilicus is more cosmetically pleasing that was prior to the surgery.

I often joke that I leave belly buttons "25% cuter" than I found them. Scars are never visible but, occasionally, healing will change an "innie" to an "outie" or a rare patient will have some less than perfect cosmesis. I have seen few of these in my career.

One other pearl that I need to include here is that I would recommend putting a Band-Aid™ on the incisions, not Steri-Strips or surgical dressings. Band-Aids™ provide a strong placebo effect that is necessary for a patient to feel as if they have had a minor procedure, not one of the most major surgeries a woman can receive. Another small pearl is to be sure to apply the Band-Aids™ to the umbilicus while the glue is still wet. A very small percentage of patients, often in unfortunate life circumstances, have the tendency to pick at incisions or obsessively clean incisions until bleeding or redness ensues. Invariably, patients then present to the emergency room to show emergency room physicians what a horrible job you have done with their recent surgery. A Band-Aid™ that is firmly affixed to the incision with Dermabond™ glue is much less likely to befall these events, as messing with the incision will not give the patient any visual results and will likely cause pain because the Band-Aid™ is glued in place. The glue generally hardens and releases around the second day postoperatively, which is when I recommend patients remove the bandages in the shower. A small, remaining cone of purple glue will then fall out over the next week, or be removed during the first postoperative appointment.

References:

62) Helgstrand, F., Rosenberg, J., & Bisgaard, T. (2011). Trocar site hernia after laparoscopic surgery: a qualitative systematic review. Hernia, 15(2), 113-121.
63) Karthik, S., Augustine, A. J., Shibumon, M. M., & Pai, M. V. (2013). Analysis of laparoscopic port site complications: A descriptive study. Journal of minimal access surgery, 9(2), 59.
64) McMurrick, P. J., & Polglase, A. L. (1993). Early incisional hernia after use of the 12 mm port for laparoscopic surgery. Australian and New Zealand Journal of Surgery, 63(7), 574-575.
65) Singal, R., Zaman, M., Mittal, A., Singal, S., Sandhu, K., & Mittal, A. (2016). No need of fascia closure to reduce trocar site hernia rate in laparoscopic surgery: a prospective study of 200 non-obese patients. Gastroenterology research, 9(4-5), 70.
66) Elashry, O. M., Nakada, S. Y., Wolf, J. J., Figenshau, R. S., McDougall, E. M., & Clayman, R. V. (1996). Comparative clinical study of port-closure techniques following laparoscopic surgery. Journal of the American College of Surgeons, 183(4), 335-344.

Chapter 14

The Horrible Way the World will end if you Don't see Jets in the Bladder

"A long habit of not thinking a thing wrong gives it a superficial appearance of being right."

- Thomas Paine

If you're reading this book, odds are on you've been there. You were performing an extremely difficult laparoscopic hysterectomy. If it was robotic, maybe it was single port but, regardless, the uterus was large, the adhesions were intense, and of course anesthesia would not give you the Trendelenburg you needed. You fought for an hour, maybe several hours with the adhesions and with the uterus, or maybe you weren't even the surgeon. Maybe you were the assistant and you watched your colleague nobly fight against adhesions, takedown difficult pedicles, and sometimes make 3 or 4 attempts to quell each bleeding vessel. Maybe the bladder was retro-filled 10 or 20 times, maybe 4 or 5 accessory 5 mm ports were placed to get the right angle. Following all of this, a ureteral injury was detected and ***a urologist you had never met made a large vertical midline incision, effectively destroying all of your hard work***. If you have had your corn flakes shit in this way, odds are you are just a little bit anxious about the possibility of a ureteral injury following hysterectomy.

Many others have described different techniques for detecting a ureteral injury at time of hysterectomy.[66] I cannot take the time to discuss every single technique that has ever been attempted to detect a ureteral injury or to prevent one, but there are a few techniques that are worth mentioning. First of all, if you routinely have the urology service place lit ureteral stents prior to performing your hysterectomies, you probably should not be performing hysterectomies. Stents, even when placed by expert urologists, have complication rates. Stents should not be used with simple, benign procedures and, although the occasional extremely adhesed hysterectomy will require stents, it should not be the M.O. for anyone receiving a hysterectomy.

While I am a fan of cystoscopy at the end of a hysterectomy, I am not necessarily one of those who feels you need to inject intravenous medicines into the patient in order to see the jets of urine. These substances, whether indigo carmine, methylene blue, or oral Pyridium, invariably have an amount of time before they will appear in the urine, and an equally unpredictable amount of time until they will cease to affect the urine. Therefore, their usefulness is limited. A good alternative is a direct injection of dextrose into the bladder. Sugary dextrose gives the fluid in the bladder clear visibility, especially urine from the ureteral orifices. It can be injected moments before cystoscopy directly into the bladder, clamping the distal portion of the Foley catheter and injecting the dextrose before removing the catheter. The best part is, it does not require any waiting whatsoever, therefore its utility is more predictable.[67]

So do I recommend cystoscopy after every hysterectomy? Yes. Not as much for the ureters as for the bladder. After decades of hysterectomies, I realized that the edge of the bladder can appear in a lot of places you would not predict. Therefore, I think the safest course of action is to perform a quick cystoscopy to make sure there are no defects in the bladder. If one fails to identify a defect in the bladder, the absence of a Foley catheter will make it essentially impossible for the defect to heal. This will certainly crash back into your E.R. with embarrassing results. But, as far as checking the ureters for jets of urine after every hysterectomy, I am not entirely sure that this is necessary, especially in light of the focus of this technique.

The focus of this entire technique is to avoid the areas where the ureter could be. Therefore, if I really feel that this technique is effective, it really does not make sense for me to advocate the routine monitoring of jets of urine following the procedure. What I do advocate, however, is the careful reasoning of your current clinical scenario before performing the cystoscopy.

It is clear when you are performing the cystoscopy following this hysterectomy that you are going to need to think about the possibility of a bladder injury. As you are definitely going to be looking for a bladder injury at time of cystoscopy, you do not need to think about it beforehand. What we really need to do is take a few seconds and think hard about how well you faithfully performed this procedure.

The real question is: how long am I willing to wait to see urine jets? In the event that you have faithfully performed this procedure avoiding the bladder and at no time were the jaws of your bipolar device in close proximity to the sidewalls, I would say you really have nothing to worry about at time of cystoscopy. I would say there is no reason to wait around for jets of urine from the ureteral orifices, and that a quick cystoscopy in order to rule out the possibility of a cystotomy is all that's required.

In fact, it can be comforting for some surgeons to tell the operating room staff that they're really only worried about a cystotomy and that is the only reason they are doing the hysterectomy. This will certainly get them off the hook, as many other surgeons in the hospital probably perform long cystoscopies waiting for jets of urine from both ureteral orifices.

In the event that you are not so certain that you've been loyal to the adherence of the technique of this procedure, consideration should be given for what exactly your guidelines are for what you are going to do before you begin the cystoscopy. If you are so worried about a ureteral injury that you are willing to watch until you see a jet of urine, up to an hour if need be, and then you plan to call a urologist to come over the operating room right then if you do not, then you need to internalize that anxiety prior to performing the cystoscopy. Do not let the staff that is anxious to leave or the impatient nurse prepping your next patient change your mind.

In most cases, experienced surgeons should rely on the premise that they are doubtful of the possibility of ureteral injury and are planning to watch the ureteral site, perhaps incidentally, for a small time. This watching is in the hopes that they will see a jet of urine for some type of "bonus" reassurance. In most patients, however, if you have faithfully performed this procedure, there is no reason to wait for the jets of urine.

Please do not miss the point that this needs to be decided ahead of time. The operating room staff is not going to let you abandon a cystoscopy 10 minutes into it if you have been waiting for degenerative urine and there is no evidence of it. The majority of the time, when you can't see the jet, it is actually just the result of dehydration, and under even more rare circumstances that the ureter may not have produced a strong jet of urine for years.

Nonetheless, you could be stuck for hours waiting for a jet of urine while the operating room staff quietly watches, judging you for your poor surgical skills that clearly caused a serious complication. So think it through ahead of time.

I cannot overstate the importance of having your certain criteria for when you will abort a cystoscopy right before you begin the procedure. If there is no doubt in your mind that the ureters were not injured at time of hysterectomy there is simply no reason for a 1 hour cystoscopy in order to see a small jet of urine from the left ureter that may not have functioned well to begin with.

In conclusion, waiting around for jets of urine from bilateral ureteral orifices is a waste of time for those faithfully performing this technique and should be reserved for the very rare scenario where a serious departure from the techniques described in this text is required. I would also say that going into a cystoscopy with a requirement that you need to see jets of urine from both ureters etc. is a vanishingly rare scenario that should only be experienced once or twice during an experienced surgeon's lifetime.

The more common scenario should be that a surgeon would feel greatly relieved by seeing a jet of urine from one particular ureteral orifice, but accepts that it is not worth the possibility of waiting up to half an hour to 2 hours of cystoscopy in order to see that checked. It should be a very rare occurrence that an experienced surgeon insists on prolonged cystoscopy to see a jet of urine from both sides.

Is it the end of the world if ureteral injury goes unidentified and the ureteral implantation has to take place on another day? Probably not.

Especially if the only way to fix the injury at time of hysterectomy would have been an open procedure, there is really not much lost. Still, standard of care dictates that if ureteral injury is suspected, immediate repair should be arranged for. The patient should not be forced to have a second surgery. This should be kept in mind, but I would reemphasize that the most important part of this discussion is that the surgeon takes the time to have a clear picture of what they hope to accomplish by performing the cystoscopy following the hysterectomy, and under what circumstances they will terminate the cystoscopy and feel comfortable enough to wake the patient.

I would wager that if you are faithfully performing this procedure, for a competent surgeon the majority of cystoscopies should be terminated with the simple reassurance that you have been able to visualize that there is no evidence of cystotomy.

References:

67) Wu, H. H., Yang, P. Y., Yeh, G. P., Chou, P. H., Hsu, J. C., & Lin, K. C. (2006). The detection of ureteral injuries after hysterectomy. Journal of minimally invasive gynecology, 13(5), 403-408.

68) Siff, L. N., Unger, C. A., Jelovsek, J. E., Paraiso, M. F. R., Ridgeway, B. M., & Barber, M. D. (2016). Assessing ureteral patency using 10% dextrose cystoscopy fluid: evaluation of urinary tract infection rates. American journal of obstetrics and gynecology, 215(1), 74-e1.

Chapter 15

La Fin - And A Very Open Invitation

So here we are, back at the Inn of the Last Home, enjoying Otik's spiced potatoes. As for the post-operative counseling, there's not much. They can stay overnight or go home after the spinal wears off. Most hospitals like outpatient hysterectomy programs, just be sure they have the right kind of spinal anesthesia if you expect the patient's legs to work when they get home. I see all surgical patients within a week and strongly encourage stool softeners and decreased activity. Of course, the only absolutely contraindicated action is objects in the vagina.

I certainly hope this journey has been educational and entertaining to you. Hopefully, it was of some value. The fact that you have finished reading this entire book qualifies you as a level-headed, knowledge-driven person who is not easily offended or upset. I am proud to have you as a colleague. Therefore, if you have taken the time to read this text and hear all my crazy opinions, I would love to hear yours. I would appreciate all feedback on this technique - especially negative feedback.

My hope is that a lot of surgeons will be comforted by the peculiar way in which this book reads and gives you insight into the mind of a surgeon doing pretty much what you do every day.

I will leave you with the same notion that I started this book with: please use this technique to the best of your ability to help as many patients as you can.

Thank you!

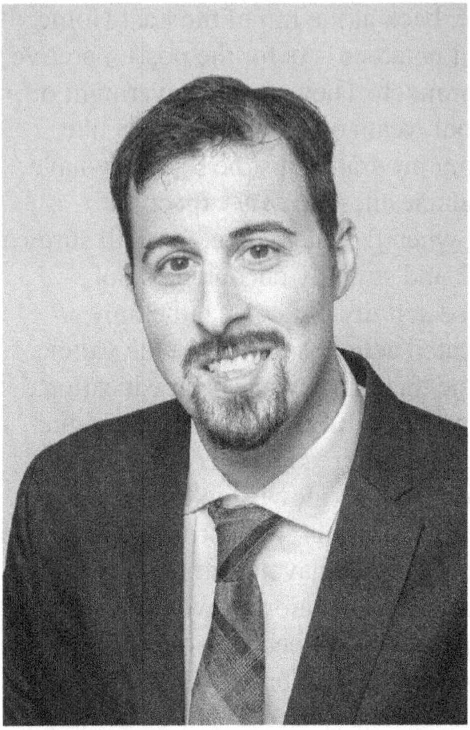

About the Author: Dr. Marchand is originally from Providence, RI, and is a board certified physician in Obstetrics and Gynecology. Dr. Marchand completed training in Obstetrics and Gynecology at the University of Tennessee, and is extensively published in the field of Minimally Invasive Surgery. Dr. Marchand is the Director of the Marchand Institute for Minimally Invasive Surgery in Mesa, Arizona, a not-for-profit surgical research and education think tank dedicated to improving minimally invasive surgery for women in the US. In addition to research and education, the institute also hosts accredited fellowship programs in Minimally Invasive Gynecologic Surgery. Dr. Marchand is recognized internationally as a pioneer in developing laparoscopic techniques, as well as an expert minimally invasive surgeon and teaching surgeon. Dr. Marchand holds several Surgical World Records, and was recently honored with a World Record for performing a total laparoscopic hysterectomy thought the smallest incision ever. Dr. Marchand was also one half of the team that was recognized by the Guinness Book of World Records™ for removing a seven pound uterus without needing to cut open the patient.

Dr. Marchand was the first surgeon in Arizona to receive the "Master Surgeon" designation from the Surgical Review Corporation™ and is also currently one of only a few accredited Master Surgeons in Minimally Invasive Gynecology in the USA. In addition, Dr. Marchand is one of the few OBGYN's in the country to be a fellow of both ACOG (American College of Obstetrics and Gynecology) and ACS (American College of Surgeons.) Dr. Marchand frequently appears in the mainstream media as an expert, and has appeared on Inside Edition™ and The Today Show™ for expert opinions in Obstetrics and Gynecology. When he is not in the operating room, Dr. Marchand enjoys low carb living and chasing around his six year old son, Sebastian.

Made in the USA
Monee, IL
14 September 2026

63198315R00069